Introduction:

Honey, the golden nectar produced by industrious bees, is more than just a sweet indulgence for your taste buds. Beyond its delightful flavor, honey has been cherished for centuries for its remarkable versatility and numerous health benefits. From its natural sweetness to its therapeutic properties, honey proves to be a multifaceted substance that goes far beyond being a simple sweetener. In this exploration, we'll delve into the myriad ways in which honey can enhance your well-being, from its nutritional richness to its healing properties. So, let's uncover the fascinating world of honey and discover how this ancient elixir can do wonders for you.

What is the difference between honey and floral honey?

"Honey" is a broad term that refers to the sweet, viscous substance produced by bees using nectar from flowers. It is a natural sweetener that has been used by humans for centuries. The term "floral honey" is often used to specify the type of honey based on the predominant source of nectar gathered by bees. Here are the key differences between honey and floral honey:

Honey:

1. **Definition:**
   - "Honey" is a general term for the sweet substance produced by bees through the collection and transformation of nectar.
2. **Production:**
   - Bees collect nectar from a variety of flowering plants and bring it back to the hive.
   - The nectar is then mixed with enzymes in the bee's saliva and stored in honeycombs.
   - Through a process of evaporation and enzymatic activity, the nectar is transformed into honey.
3. **Varieties:**
   - Honey comes in various varieties, each with its own unique flavor, color, and aroma.
   - The taste of honey can be influenced by the types of flowers the bees visited to collect nectar.

Floral Honey:

1. **Definition:**
   - "Floral honey" is a term used to describe honey that predominantly comes from the

nectar of specific flowers or a particular type of plant.

2. **Varieties:**
   - Different varieties of floral honey are named based on the primary floral source. For example:
     - **Clover Honey:** Comes from the nectar of clover flowers.
     - **Orange Blossom Honey:** Comes from the nectar of orange blossom flowers.
     - **Lavender Honey:** Comes from the nectar of lavender flowers.
     - **Acacia Honey:** Comes from the nectar of acacia flowers.
   - The specific floral source influences the taste, color, and aroma of the honey.

3. **Characteristics:**
   - Floral honey can have distinct characteristics based on the types of flowers the bees visited.
   - The flavor profile may range from mild and light to robust and intense.

Key Points:

- **All Floral Honey is Honey:**

- All floral honey is a type of honey, but not all honey is necessarily specified as "floral honey."
- **Geographical Influence:**
  - The geographical location and climate can also influence the types of flowers available to bees and, consequently, the floral honey produced in a specific region.
- **Single-Source vs. Multifloral:**
  - Floral honey can be single-source (from one predominant flower type) or multifloral (a blend of nectars from various flowers).
- **Labeling:**
  - When you see honey labeled with a specific flower name (e.g., "Wildflower Honey"), it implies a mixture of nectars from various flowers rather than a single floral source.

In summary, while "honey" is the general term for the sweet substance produced by bees, "floral honey" specifies the type of honey based on the predominant floral source. The distinction is made to highlight the unique flavors and characteristics that result from the diverse array of flowers bees visit to collect nectar.

How do you harvest honey?

Harvesting honey involves collecting mature, capped honeycombs from beehives. This process is typically done by beekeepers who manage honeybee colonies. Here are the general steps involved in harvesting honey:

1. Assessing Hive Readiness:

- **Maturity of Honey:**
    - Ensure that the honey in the hive is mature and capped. Capped cells indicate that the honey has been properly processed and is ready for harvest.
- **Seasonal Timing:**
    - Harvesting is usually done during the honey flow season when nectar is abundant, and bees are actively collecting and storing it.

2. Gathering Equipment:

- **Protective Gear:**
    - Wear appropriate beekeeping protective gear, including a bee suit, veil, gloves, and boots, to minimize the risk of stings.
- **Bee Smoker:**
    - Use a bee smoker to calm the bees before opening the hive.
- **Hive Tool:**
    - Have a hive tool to pry apart hive components and lift frames.

3. Preparing the Hive:

- **Smoking the Hive:**
  - Use the bee smoker to produce smoke at the hive entrance and within the hive. This helps calm the bees, making them less defensive.
- **Removing Bees:**
  - Gently brush or blow bees off the honey frames to minimize the number of bees present during the harvest.

4. Removing Frames:

- **Inspecting Frames:**
  - Inspect each frame to ensure that the honey is capped, indicating its maturity.
- **Uncapping Honey:**
  - If not using an extractor, the honeycomb cells need to be uncapped using a hot knife, uncapping fork, or other tools. This exposes the honey for extraction.

5. Extracting Honey:

- **Honey Extractor:**
  - Place the frames in a honey extractor—a device that uses centrifugal force to spin honey out of the cells.

- **Uncapping Tank:**
    - If frames were manually uncapped, place them over an uncapping tank to collect the released honey.

6. Filtering and Settling:

- **Filtering Honey:**
    - Filter the extracted honey to remove debris, wax particles, and air bubbles. This can be done using fine mesh or cheesecloth.
- **Settling:**
    - Allow the filtered honey to settle in a container for some time. This helps air bubbles rise to the top, and any remaining impurities settle.

7. Bottling:

- **Bottling Honey:**
    - Transfer the clear honey into jars or other storage containers. Use a honey gate or a funnel to make the process more manageable.

8. Storing and Labeling:

- **Storing Jars:**

- Store honey in a cool, dry place. Avoid exposure to direct sunlight or excessive heat.
- **Labeling:**
    - Label each jar with the date of harvest, floral source (if known), and any other relevant information.

9. Returning Frames to the Hive:

- **Returning Empty Frames:**
    - Return the frames to the hive for the bees to clean and reuse. Bees will remove any remaining honey and cap the cells for storage.

Tips:

- **Consider Extraction Methods:**
    - Besides honey extractors, some beekeepers use crush-and-strain methods, where they crush the honeycomb and strain the honey. This method requires more effort but is an alternative for those without extractors.
- **Work Efficiently:**
    - Harvest honey efficiently to minimize the disruption to the hive and reduce stress on the bees.
- **Leave Sufficient Honey for Bees:**

- Always leave enough honey in the hive for the bees to sustain themselves through the winter or periods of low nectar flow.
- **Regular Inspections:**
  - Regular hive inspections and proper hive management contribute to a healthy colony and a successful honey harvest.

It's important to note that beekeeping and honey harvesting should be done with care and consideration for the well-being of the bees. Additionally, local regulations and guidelines may apply, so beekeepers should be aware of and adhere to any relevant beekeeping laws and practices in their area.

How do you build a bee hive?

Building a beehive is a rewarding project for those interested in beekeeping. Here's a basic guide on how to build a Langstroth-style beehive, one of the most common hive designs used by beekeepers:

Materials Needed:

1. **Lumber:**
   - Select high-quality, untreated wood. Cedar or pine are commonly used.
   - Typical hive components are made from 3/4-inch thick wood.

2. **Tools:**
    - Table saw or circular saw
    - Miter saw
    - Electric drill
    - Wood glue
    - Wood screws
    - Clamps
    - Hive tool (for prying apart frames)
3. **Hardware:**
    - Nails or screws (galvanized or stainless steel to resist rust)
    - Hive entrance reducer
    - Hive stand or bottom board
    - Inner cover
    - Outer cover
    - Frames and foundation

Steps to Build a Langstroth Beehive:

1. Assemble the Hive Stand or Bottom Board:

- Cut the bottom board to the desired dimensions.
- Attach cleats to elevate the hive slightly for ventilation.
- Attach a landing board at the entrance.

2. Build the Deep Hive Body (Brood Box):

- Cut the front, back, and side panels for the deep hive body.

- Assemble the panels using wood glue and screws.
- Install handles on the sides for easy lifting.

3. Add Frames and Foundation to the Deep Hive Body:

- Insert wooden frames with wax foundation into the deep hive body.
- Frames should be spaced evenly.

4. Add the Queen Excluder (Optional):

- If using a queen excluder, place it on top of the deep hive body.

5. Build the Medium Hive Bodies (Supers):

- Follow the same process as for the deep hive body to create medium hive bodies.
- Medium supers are where bees store surplus honey.

6. Add Frames and Foundation to the Medium Hive Bodies:

- Insert frames with wax foundation into the medium hive bodies.
- Ensure frames are evenly spaced.

7. Assemble the Inner Cover:

- Create an inner cover by attaching a wooden frame to a plywood board.

- Drill a hole in the center for ventilation.

8. Build the Outer Cover:

- Construct the outer cover using plywood and a wooden frame.
- Add a telescoping cover for weather protection.

9. Paint or Seal the Components:

- Paint or seal the hive components to protect the wood from the elements.
- Use non-toxic paint or sealant to avoid harming the bees.

10. Assemble the Components:

- Stack the components in the following order from the bottom up:
    1. Hive stand or bottom board
    2. Deep hive body (brood box)
    3. Queen excluder (if used)
    4. Medium hive bodies (supers)
    5. Inner cover
    6. Outer cover

11. Add Bees and Frames:

- Once the hive is assembled, introduce a package of bees or a nucleus colony.
- Insert frames with foundation into the deep hive body and medium hive bodies.

12. Maintain and Monitor:

- Regularly inspect the hive, monitor hive health, and conduct routine maintenance.

Additional Tips:

- **Follow Hive Dimensions:**
    - Use standard Langstroth hive dimensions for compatibility with commercially available frames and foundation.
- **Safety First:**
    - Wear appropriate protective gear, including gloves and a bee suit, when working with bees.
- **Educate Yourself:**
    - Familiarize yourself with beekeeping practices and consider taking a local beekeeping course.
- **Local Regulations:**
    - Check local regulations regarding beekeeping and hive placement.

Building a beehive requires precision and attention to detail, so take your time during the construction process. Additionally, consider reaching out to local beekeeping associations or mentors for guidance and support as you start your beekeeping journey.

How do you attract bees to your beehive?

Attracting bees to your beehive involves creating an environment that is appealing to honeybees and providing them with the necessary conditions to establish and thrive in a hive. Here are some steps to attract bees to your beehive:

1. Choose a Suitable Location:

- **Sun Exposure:**
    - Select a location that receives ample sunlight, preferably facing south or southeast. Bees are more active in warmer, sunny conditions.
- **Protection from Wind:**
    - Provide some protection from strong winds, as bees prefer a sheltered environment.
- **Accessible Water Source:**
    - Ensure there is a clean and accessible water source near the hive for the bees. Bees need water for cooling the hive and diluting honey for consumption.

2. Use Bee-Friendly Plants:

- **Plant Bee-Friendly Flowers:**

- Surround the hive with a variety of bee-friendly plants that produce nectar and pollen. Flowers like lavender, sunflowers, clover, and bee balm are attractive to bees.
- **Create a Bee Garden:**
    - Design a bee garden with a mix of flowers that bloom throughout the seasons. This provides a continuous food source for the bees.

3. Provide a Water Source:

- **Shallow Water Container:**
    - Place a shallow container with water near the hive. Add floating objects like cork or stones to provide bees a safe platform to land on while drinking.

4. Use Pheromones and Attractants:

- **Lure Swarm Attractants:**
    - Consider using commercially available swarm attractants that mimic the pheromones released by a queen bee. These attractants can be used to lure swarms to an empty hive.

5. Utilize Bait Hives:

- **Set Up Bait Hives:**

- Bait hives are empty hives placed strategically to attract swarming bees. They are typically set up in the early spring when swarming is more likely.
- **Add Old Comb or Lure:**
  - Place old comb or commercially available lures in the bait hive to make it more attractive to scout bees.

6. Establish a Nucleus Colony:

- **Purchase a Nucleus (Nuc) Colony:**
  - Acquire a small nucleus colony from a reputable source. Nucleus colonies are smaller, established bee colonies with a queen, workers, and brood.

7. Maintain a Clean and Dry Hive:

- **Clean Equipment:**
  - Ensure that your beehive equipment is clean and free from old comb or debris.
- **Ventilation:**
  - Provide proper hive ventilation to maintain a dry and comfortable environment for the bees.

8. Be Patient:

- **Allow Time:**

- Bees are naturally attracted to suitable hive conditions. Sometimes, it takes time for scout bees to discover a new hive, so be patient.

9. Use Swarm Lures (Optional):

- **Commercial Swarm Lures:**
  - Some beekeepers use commercially available swarm lures that mimic the scent of a queen bee. These lures can attract swarms to a new hive.

10. Seek Local Advice:

- **Consult Local Beekeepers:**
  - Seek advice from local beekeepers who are familiar with the specific conditions in your area. They may provide valuable insights into attracting bees to your hive.

Important Considerations:

- **Avoid Pesticides:**
  - Avoid using pesticides or herbicides near the hive, as they can harm bees.
- **Adhere to Regulations:**
  - Ensure compliance with local regulations and zoning ordinances related to beekeeping.

- **Consider Professional Help:**
  - If you're new to beekeeping, consider seeking the assistance of experienced beekeepers or mentors.

By creating an attractive and suitable environment, providing food sources, and being patient, you increase the chances of attracting bees to your beehive. Always prioritize the well-being of the bees and follow sustainable and ethical beekeeping practices.

Does lemon-balm attract bees?

Yes, lemon balm (Melissa officinalis) is known to attract bees. Lemon balm is a fragrant herb with a lemony scent, and its small white or pale yellow flowers produce nectar that is attractive to bees. Bees are particularly drawn to plants that offer nectar and pollen, and lemon balm is considered a bee-friendly plant.

If you are interested in attracting bees to your garden or beekeeping area, planting lemon balm can be a beneficial addition. Bees play a crucial role in pollination, and providing them with a variety of nectar-rich plants helps support their foraging and contributes to the health of local bee populations.

When cultivating lemon balm for bee attraction, here are some tips:

1. **Planting:** Plant lemon balm in a sunny location with well-drained soil. It's a hardy herb that can grow well in various conditions.
2. **Companion Planting:** Consider planting lemon balm alongside other bee-friendly plants to create a diverse and attractive environment for pollinators.
3. **Harvesting:** While lemon balm is known for its aromatic leaves, you can also allow some of the plants to flower to provide a nectar source for bees. Bees are attracted not only to the fragrance of the leaves but also to the flowers.
4. **Avoid Pesticides:** To ensure a safe and healthy environment for bees, avoid using pesticides or herbicides that could harm them.

Remember that providing a variety of flowering plants throughout the growing season is beneficial for attracting and supporting bees. Bee-friendly gardens contribute to the overall health of local ecosystems and promote biodiversity.

What flowers should you plant to make the best honey?

To produce the best honey, it's essential to plant a variety of flowers that provide bees with a diverse and abundant source of nectar. The flavor, aroma, and characteristics of honey are influenced by the types of flowers the bees visit. Here are some flowers that are known to produce high-quality and flavorful honey:

1. **Clover (Trifolium spp.):**
   - White clover and alsike clover are common sources of honey. Clover honey is light and mild with a sweet taste.
2. **Lavender (Lavandula spp.):**
   - Lavender produces a fragrant honey with a distinct floral aroma and a slightly sweet and herbal flavor.
3. **Acacia (Robinia pseudoacacia):**
   - Acacia honey is prized for its light color, mild flavor, and slow crystallization. It is often considered one of the best honeys.
4. **Citrus Blossoms (Citrus spp.):**
   - Orange blossom honey, lemon blossom honey, and other citrus blossom honeys have a citrusy aroma and a sweet, fruity flavor.
5. **Basswood or Linden (Tilia spp.):**
   - Linden honey has a light color, pleasant aroma, and a delicate, slightly minty or woody flavor.
6. **Alfalfa (Medicago sativa):**

- Alfalfa honey is light amber in color and has a mild, slightly floral taste.

7. **Sunflower (Helianthus spp.):**
   - Sunflower honey is golden in color with a mild, buttery flavor.

8. **Buckwheat (Fagopyrum esculentum):**
   - Buckwheat honey is dark and robust with a strong, molasses-like flavor. It's known for its antioxidant properties.

9. **Wildflowers:**
   - Planting a mix of native wildflowers provides a diverse range of nectar sources and contributes to the complexity of the honey's flavor.

10. **Blueberry (Vaccinium spp.):**
    - Blueberry honey has a distinctive fruity flavor with hints of blueberry. It's often dark amber to reddish-brown in color.

11. **Manuka (Leptospermum scoparium):**
    - Manuka honey is produced from the nectar of the manuka tree in New Zealand. It has unique medicinal properties and a strong, earthy flavor.

12. **Heather (Calluna vulgaris and Erica spp.):**
    - Heather honey is dark and has a strong, distinctive flavor. It's often described as robust and slightly bitter.

When planning a garden or apiary for honey production, aim for a mix of early, mid-season, and late-blooming plants to provide a continuous nectar flow throughout the growing season. Additionally, local conditions and climate can influence which plants thrive in your area and are attractive to bees. Consulting with local beekeeping experts or agricultural extension services can provide valuable insights into the best flower varieties for honey production in your specific region.

Is honey good for your skin?

Yes, honey is often considered beneficial for the skin due to its various properties that promote skin health. Here are some ways in which honey can be good for your skin:

1. **Moisturizing:** Honey is a natural humectant, which means it attracts and retains moisture. Applying honey to your skin can help keep it hydrated, making it an excellent ingredient for moisturizing masks.
2. **Antioxidant Properties:** Honey contains antioxidants that help protect the skin from damage caused by free radicals. This can contribute to maintaining skin's elasticity and overall youthful appearance.

3. **Anti-Inflammatory:** Honey possesses anti-inflammatory properties, which can be beneficial for soothing and calming irritated or inflamed skin. It may help alleviate conditions such as acne or redness.
4. **Wound Healing:** Honey has been used for centuries as a natural remedy for wound healing. Its antimicrobial properties can help prevent infections, and it creates a protective barrier over wounds, promoting faster healing.
5. **Acne Treatment:** The antibacterial properties of honey can be beneficial for individuals dealing with acne. Applying honey to acne-prone areas may help reduce bacteria and inflammation.
6. **Exfoliation:** Honey can act as a gentle exfoliant, helping to remove dead skin cells and promote a smoother complexion. Mixing honey with other natural ingredients like oats or yogurt can enhance its exfoliating properties.
7. **Scar Fading:** Regular use of honey on scars may contribute to their gradual fading over time. The wound-healing and regenerative properties of honey can aid in minimizing the appearance of scars.

When using honey for skincare, it's advisable to choose raw, unprocessed honey as it retains more of its beneficial properties. Additionally, conducting a patch test before applying honey to a larger area can help ensure that you do not have any adverse reactions.

While honey can be a valuable addition to your skincare routine, it's essential to complement it with a well-rounded skincare regimen and consult with a dermatologist for specific skin concerns.

Unprocessed honey vs store bought honey

The main difference between unprocessed honey and store-bought honey lies in their production and processing methods. Here's a breakdown of the distinctions:

1. **Raw or Unprocessed Honey:**
   - **Production:** Raw honey is directly extracted from the honeycomb and is not heated or processed. It is essentially honey in its most natural form.
   - **Texture and Appearance:** Raw honey often has a cloudy or crystallized appearance, as it contains particles and remnants of beeswax.
   - **Flavor:** The flavor profile of raw honey can vary significantly depending on the flowers from which the bees collected nectar. It is often considered more flavorful and robust compared to processed honey.
   - **Nutrient Content:** Raw honey retains more of its natural vitamins, enzymes,

antioxidants, and other beneficial compounds due to minimal processing.

2. **Store-Bought or Processed Honey:**
    - **Production:** Commercially available honey often undergoes processing, including pasteurization and filtration. Pasteurization involves heating the honey to eliminate yeast and prevent crystallization.
    - **Texture and Appearance:** Processed honey is usually clear and liquid, with a smooth texture. It may remain in this state for a longer time due to pasteurization.
    - **Flavor:** Processed honey may have a milder taste compared to raw honey, as the heating process can alter the flavor and aroma.
    - **Nutrient Content:** Processing methods can result in the loss of some beneficial enzymes, vitamins, and antioxidants found in raw honey. However, honey still retains many of its health benefits even after processing.

When choosing between raw and processed honey, it often comes down to personal preference and intended use. Some people prefer the distinct flavor and potential health benefits of raw honey, while others may opt for the convenience and longer shelf life of processed honey.

It's worth noting that both types of honey can be enjoyed and used in various ways, such as sweetening beverages, drizzling over food, or incorporating into recipes. If you're specifically seeking the potential health benefits associated with raw honey, it's advisable to look for honey labeled as "raw" or "unprocessed" and sourced from reputable sources.

How do you use honey for your skin? Is there a specific way to use it? Is there a recipe?

Using honey for your skin is relatively simple, and there are various ways to incorporate it into your skincare routine. Here are some common methods and a simple recipe:

1. **Honey Mask:**
    - **Ingredients:**
        - 1-2 tablespoons of raw honey
        - Optional: A few drops of lemon juice, yogurt, or aloe vera gel (for additional benefits)
    - **Instructions:**
        1. Cleanse your face to remove any makeup or impurities.
        2. Apply a thin layer of raw honey evenly to your face.
        3. Leave the honey mask on for 15-20 minutes.

    4. Rinse your face thoroughly with warm water.

    5. Pat your face dry with a clean towel.

This mask can help moisturize, soothe, and rejuvenate your skin. The optional ingredients can be customized based on your skin type and needs.

2. **Spot Treatment for Acne:**
   - Apply a small amount of raw honey directly to acne spots or blemishes.
   - Leave it on for 15-20 minutes.
   - Rinse off with warm water.

The antibacterial properties of honey can be beneficial for treating acne.

3. **Exfoliating Honey Scrub:**
   - **Ingredients:**
     - 1 tablespoon of raw honey
     - 1 tablespoon of fine sugar or ground oats
   - **Instructions:**
     1. Mix the honey and sugar or ground oats to create a paste.
     2. Gently massage the mixture onto your face in circular motions.
     3. Rinse off with warm water.

This exfoliating scrub helps remove dead skin cells, leaving your skin feeling smooth.

4. **Hydrating Honey Bath:**

- Add 2 tablespoons of raw honey to your bathwater.
- Soak in the bath for 15-20 minutes.
- Pat your skin dry after the bath.

This can help moisturize and soften your skin.

Remember to do a patch test before using honey on your face, especially if you have sensitive skin, to ensure you don't have any adverse reactions. Also, choose raw, unprocessed honey for maximum benefits. Additionally, if you have specific skin concerns, it's a good idea to consult with a dermatologist before incorporating new ingredients into your skincare routine.

Is Honey beneficial for your hair? How do you use it?

Yes, honey can be beneficial for your hair in several ways. It is known for its moisturizing, conditioning, and nourishing properties. Here are some ways you can use honey for your hair:

1. **Hair Mask for Moisture:**
   - **Ingredients:**
     - 2 tablespoons of raw honey
     - 1-2 tablespoons of coconut oil or olive oil
   - **Instructions:**

1. Mix the honey and oil in a bowl until well combined.
2. Apply the mixture to damp hair, starting from the roots to the tips.
3. Cover your hair with a shower cap and leave the mask on for 20-30 minutes.
4. Rinse thoroughly with water and shampoo as usual.

This honey and oil mask can help moisturize and hydrate dry or damaged hair.

2. **Honey and Apple Cider Vinegar Rinse:**
   - **Ingredients:**
     - 1-2 tablespoons of raw honey
     - 1 cup of water
     - 1-2 tablespoons of apple cider vinegar
   - **Instructions:**
     1. Mix the honey, water, and apple cider vinegar in a bowl.
     2. After shampooing, pour the mixture over your hair and scalp.
     3. Massage your scalp and hair for a few minutes.
     4. Rinse your hair thoroughly with water.

This rinse can help clarify the hair, promote shine, and balance the scalp's pH.

3. **Honey and Yogurt Hair Mask:**

- **Ingredients:**
  - 2 tablespoons of raw honey
  - 1/2 cup of plain yogurt
- **Instructions:**
  1. Mix the honey and yogurt in a bowl until smooth.
  2. Apply the mixture to clean, damp hair.
  3. Cover your hair with a shower cap and leave the mask on for 20-30 minutes.
  4. Rinse thoroughly with water and shampoo as usual.

This mask can help condition the hair and provide it with essential nutrients.

4. **Honey and Aloe Vera Hair Treatment:**
   - **Ingredients:**
     - 2 tablespoons of raw honey
     - 1-2 tablespoons of aloe vera gel
   - **Instructions:**
     1. Mix the honey and aloe vera gel in a bowl.
     2. Apply the mixture to damp hair, focusing on the ends.
     3. Leave it on for 15-20 minutes.
     4. Rinse thoroughly with water.

This treatment can help soothe the scalp and promote healthy hair.

Remember to adjust the quantities based on the length and thickness of your hair. Additionally, it's recommended to perform a patch test before trying any new hair treatment to ensure you don't have any adverse reactions.

Can honey be used as an antibiotic? How do you use it?

Honey does have natural antibacterial properties, and it has been used for its medicinal properties for centuries. While it is not a substitute for prescription antibiotics in the treatment of serious infections, honey may be used as a topical treatment for minor wounds and burns. Here's how you can use honey as a natural antibiotic:

1. **Topical Application for Wounds:**
   - **Clean the Wound:** Before applying honey, make sure to clean the wound gently with mild soap and water.
   - **Apply Honey:** Dab a small amount of raw, unprocessed honey directly onto the wound or affected area.
   - **Cover the Wound:** If needed, cover the wound with a sterile bandage or gauze.
   - **Repeat:** Reapply honey and change the dressing regularly until the wound heals.

Honey's natural antibacterial properties can help prevent infection and promote wound healing.

2. **Honey and Turmeric Paste:**
   - **Ingredients:**
     - 1 tablespoon of raw honey
     - 1/2 teaspoon of turmeric powder
   - **Instructions:**
     1. Mix honey and turmeric powder to form a paste.
     2. Apply the paste to the affected area.
     3. Leave it on for 15-20 minutes.
     4. Rinse off with water.

Turmeric has additional anti-inflammatory properties, and combining it with honey can enhance the wound-healing effects.

3. **Honey and Lemon Gargle for Sore Throat:**
   - **Ingredients:**
     - 1 tablespoon of raw honey
     - 1 tablespoon of fresh lemon juice
   - **Instructions:**
     1. Mix honey and lemon juice in warm water to create a soothing gargle solution.
     2. Gargle with the mixture to help soothe a sore throat.

This combination can help with throat irritation and has antimicrobial properties.

While honey can be beneficial for minor wounds and sore throats, it's important to note that you should consult a healthcare professional for serious infections, and antibiotics prescribed by a doctor are necessary for bacterial infections that require systemic treatment. Additionally, people with allergies to bee products should avoid using honey topically or internally. Always use raw, unprocessed honey for these purposes, as processing may reduce its antibacterial properties.

What do microbes do in your body? How does this pertain to honey?

Microbes, which include bacteria, viruses, fungi, and other microorganisms, play crucial roles in the human body, contributing to various aspects of health and well-being. While the term "microbes" is often associated with harmful pathogens, it's essential to recognize that many microorganisms are beneficial and even necessary for the proper functioning of the body. Here's an overview of the roles of microbes in the body and how this pertains to honey:

1. **Gut Microbiota:**
    - **Role:** The human gastrointestinal tract is home to a vast community of microorganisms known as the gut microbiota. These microbes aid in

digestion, help extract nutrients from food, and contribute to the synthesis of certain vitamins.

- **Pertinence to Honey:** Some studies suggest that certain components of honey may have prebiotic properties, meaning they can support the growth and activity of beneficial bacteria in the gut. This can contribute to a healthy balance of gut microbiota.

2. **Immune System Regulation:**

   - **Role:** Microbes play a crucial role in training and modulating the immune system. Exposure to various microbes helps the immune system distinguish between harmless substances and potential threats.

   - **Pertinence to Honey:** Honey possesses natural antimicrobial properties, which can be attributed to factors such as low water content, high acidity, and the presence of hydrogen peroxide. These properties make honey a traditional remedy for wound healing and may contribute to its ability to help soothe sore throats and coughs.

3. **Skin Microbiota:**

   - **Role:** The skin is home to a diverse community of microorganisms that contribute to maintaining a protective barrier against pathogens and help regulate skin health.

- **Pertinence to Honey:** When applied topically, honey's antimicrobial properties can help prevent infections in wounds and promote skin health. It may also influence the skin microbiota in a way that supports a balanced and healthy environment.

4. **Respiratory Health:**

- **Role:** Microbes in the respiratory system contribute to maintaining a healthy respiratory microbiome, which can help protect against respiratory infections.
- **Pertinence to Honey:** Honey has been used as a remedy for respiratory issues such as coughs and sore throats. Its antimicrobial properties, along with its soothing and coating effects, may provide relief and support respiratory health.

It's important to note that while honey contains natural antimicrobial properties, it should not be considered a substitute for medical treatment when dealing with serious infections. Additionally, the impact of honey on the microbiota is an area of ongoing research, and the specific effects may vary depending on factors such as the type of honey and individual health conditions. As always, it's advisable to consult with healthcare professionals for personalized advice on health and wellness.

What is an antioxidant? How does honey help with this? How do you use honey as an antioxidant?

An antioxidant is a substance that helps prevent or slow damage to cells caused by free radicals. Free radicals are molecules produced during normal metabolic processes, and they can also be generated by exposure to factors like pollution, radiation, and tobacco smoke. These free radicals can cause oxidative stress, which, over time, may contribute to various health issues, including inflammation and chronic diseases.

Honey contains a variety of antioxidants, including polyphenols, flavonoids, and enzymes. These compounds have been shown to have potential health benefits, including reducing oxidative stress. Here's how honey can help as an antioxidant, along with ways to incorporate it into your diet:

1. **Polyphenols and Flavonoids:**
   - **Found in Honey:** Honey, especially in its raw and unprocessed form, contains polyphenols and flavonoids, which are plant-based compounds with antioxidant properties.
   - **Benefits:** These antioxidants help neutralize free radicals, reducing oxidative

stress and its potential negative impact on cells.

2. **Enzymes:**
   - **Found in Honey:** Honey contains enzymes such as glucose oxidase, which produces hydrogen peroxide. Hydrogen peroxide has antimicrobial properties and contributes to honey's antioxidant effects.
   - **Benefits:** The antimicrobial and antioxidant properties of honey make it useful for promoting overall health and supporting the immune system.

3. **Vitamins and Minerals:**
   - **Found in Honey:** Honey contains small amounts of vitamins and minerals, including vitamin C and selenium, which also contribute to its antioxidant properties.
   - **Benefits:** These nutrients play a role in neutralizing free radicals and supporting the body's defense against oxidative stress.

4. **Incorporating Honey as an Antioxidant:**
   - **Add to Beverages:** Stir a teaspoon of raw honey into your tea, warm water, or a smoothie. This not only adds natural sweetness but also provides antioxidants.
   - **Drizzle Over Food:** Use honey as a topping for yogurt, oatmeal, or fresh fruit to enhance both flavor and nutritional content.

- **Include in Salad Dressings:** Mix honey with olive oil, vinegar, and herbs to create a tasty salad dressing with added antioxidant benefits.
- **Use in Cooking:** Incorporate honey into recipes for marinades, glazes, or baking to introduce its antioxidant properties to a variety of dishes.

While honey can be a valuable addition to a diet for its antioxidant content, it's important to consume it in moderation due to its calorie and sugar content. Additionally, choosing raw and minimally processed honey ensures that you retain more of its natural antioxidants. As with any dietary changes, it's a good idea to consult with a healthcare professional, especially if you have specific health concerns or conditions.

Is honey better for you than sugar?

The comparison between honey and sugar depends on various factors, including nutritional content, sweetness, and potential health benefits. Here's a breakdown of some key differences:

1. **Nutritional Content:**
   - **Honey:** While both honey and sugar are forms of carbohydrates, honey contains small amounts of vitamins, minerals,

antioxidants, and enzymes. The exact nutritional profile can vary depending on the type of honey, but it generally provides more nutrients than refined sugar.
- **Sugar:** Refined sugar, such as white or brown sugar, is primarily composed of sucrose and lacks the additional nutrients found in honey.

2. **Sweetness:**
- **Honey:** Honey is sweeter than sugar, so you may need less of it to achieve the desired level of sweetness.
- **Sugar:** Sugar is less sweet than honey, and you may need to use more of it to match the sweetness of honey.

3. **Caloric Content:**
- **Honey:** Honey is more calorie-dense than sugar due to its higher moisture content. It contains about 64 calories per tablespoon.
- **Sugar:** Granulated sugar has about 49 calories per tablespoon.

4. **Glycemic Index:**
- **Honey:** The glycemic index of honey can vary depending on its composition. Generally, honey has a lower glycemic index than some sugars, meaning it has a slower impact on blood sugar levels.

- **Sugar:** The glycemic index of sugar is higher, leading to a more rapid increase in blood sugar levels after consumption.

5. **Antioxidants and Health Benefits:**
   - **Honey:** Honey contains antioxidants, which may provide some health benefits, including potential anti-inflammatory and immune-supporting properties. The antioxidants in honey can vary based on factors like floral source and processing methods.
   - **Sugar:** Refined sugar lacks the additional nutrients and antioxidants found in honey and is often considered empty calories.

6. **Potential Impact on Blood Sugar:**
   - **Honey:** While honey has a lower glycemic index than sugar, it still raises blood sugar levels. Individuals with diabetes or those monitoring their blood sugar should use honey in moderation.
   - **Sugar:** Sugar has a higher glycemic index, leading to a quicker spike in blood sugar levels.

In summary, honey does offer some potential nutritional benefits over refined sugar due to its antioxidant content and trace amounts of vitamins and minerals. However, it's essential to use honey in moderation, as it is still a sweetener with caloric content. Individuals with specific dietary needs, such as those managing diabetes, should consult with healthcare professionals for personalized guidance on sweetener choices. Additionally, the overall impact on health depends on the context of the entire diet and lifestyle.

How does honey lower blood pressure? How do you use it to lower blood pressure?

Honey may have potential cardiovascular benefits that could contribute to the maintenance of healthy blood pressure levels. However, it's important to note that while there is some evidence suggesting these effects, more research is needed to fully understand the mechanisms and establish specific recommendations. Here are some ways honey might be associated with lower blood pressure:

1. **Antioxidant Properties:**
   - **Honey contains antioxidants,** such as polyphenols and flavonoids, which have been linked to cardiovascular health. Antioxidants help combat oxidative stress and inflammation, factors that can contribute to high blood pressure.
2. **Nitric Oxide Production:**

- **Some studies suggest that honey may stimulate the production of nitric oxide,** a molecule that plays a role in dilating blood vessels. Enhanced vasodilation can contribute to improved blood flow and potentially lower blood pressure.

3. **Mineral Content:**
   - **Honey contains small amounts of minerals,** including potassium. Adequate potassium intake is associated with blood pressure regulation, as it helps balance sodium levels in the body.

4. **Anti-Inflammatory Effects:**
   - **Chronic inflammation is linked to hypertension.** Honey's anti-inflammatory properties may help reduce inflammation, which, in turn, could positively influence blood pressure.

While these potential benefits are intriguing, it's important to approach honey consumption as part of an overall heart-healthy lifestyle. Here are some general tips on incorporating honey into your diet:

- **Choose Raw Honey:** Opt for raw, unprocessed honey to retain its natural antioxidants and other beneficial compounds. Processing methods, such as heating and filtration, can reduce some of these properties.

- **Use as a Sweetener:** Replace refined sugars with honey in moderation when sweetening beverages, such as tea or coffee, and in recipes. Keep in mind that honey is sweeter than sugar, so you may need less of it.
- **Combine with Healthy Foods:** Drizzle honey over fruits, yogurt, or whole-grain cereals to add sweetness and flavor while also benefiting from the nutritional content of these foods.
- **Honey and Cinnamon Combination:** Some people believe that combining honey with cinnamon may have additional cardiovascular benefits. You can mix a small amount of honey with cinnamon and consume it regularly.

It's crucial to note that individual responses to dietary changes can vary, and any dietary modification should be discussed with a healthcare professional, especially for individuals with existing health conditions or those taking medications. While honey can be part of a heart-healthy diet, lifestyle factors such as regular exercise, maintaining a healthy weight, and managing stress are also essential components of blood pressure management

How do bees make honey?

The process of honey production involves the coordinated efforts of worker bees, the foraging of nectar, and the activities within the beehive. Here's a step-by-step explanation of how bees make honey:

1. **Foraging for Nectar:**
   - Worker bees, which are female bees, fly from flower to flower collecting nectar. Nectar is a sugary liquid produced by flowers, and it serves as the raw material for honey production.
   - As the bee visits flowers, it uses its proboscis (a long, tube-like tongue) to suck up the nectar.

2. **Storing Nectar in the Honey Crop:**
   - The nectar is stored in a specialized pouch called the honey crop, located in the bee's abdomen. The honey crop is a temporary storage chamber separate from the bee's stomach.

3. **Enzymatic Transformation:**
   - While the bee is transporting the nectar back to the hive, enzymes are added to the nectar in the honey crop. These enzymes start breaking down the complex sugars in the nectar into simpler sugars like glucose and fructose.

4. **Deposit into Honeycomb Cells:**
   - Once back at the hive, the foraging bee regurgitates the enzymatically transformed nectar into a cell of the honeycomb.

- Bees inside the hive then work collectively to fan the nectar with their wings, helping to reduce its water content through evaporation.

5. **Water Evaporation and Ripening:**
   - The bees continue to fan the nectar until its water content is reduced to around 17-20%. This process is crucial for the preservation and stability of honey.
   - The enzymatic action and water evaporation lead to the transformation of nectar into honey. The process is often referred to as "ripening."

6. **Capping the Honeycomb Cell:**
   - Once the honey reaches the desired consistency and water content, the worker bees cap the honeycomb cell with beeswax to seal it.

7. **Storage:**
   - The sealed honeycomb cells serve as storage containers for the honey until it is needed by the colony. Bees store honey as a food source, especially during times when nectar is scarce, such as winter.

8. **Harvesting by Beekeepers:**
   - Beekeepers, when ready to harvest honey, carefully remove the capped honeycomb frames from the beehive. They extract the honey by uncapping the cells and then use

a centrifuge to spin the honey out of the comb.

9. **Filtering and Bottling:**
   - The extracted honey may be lightly filtered to remove debris and beeswax particles. However, raw honey is minimally processed to retain its natural flavors and beneficial components.
   - The honey is then bottled and ready for consumption.

This remarkable process showcases the collective efforts of worker bees, the natural transformation of nectar into honey, and the intricate organization within the beehive. It's important to note that bees play a crucial role in pollination during their foraging activities, contributing to the reproduction of many plant species and maintaining biodiversity.

Can you eat the honeycomb? Does it have health benefits? What are they?

Yes, you can eat honeycomb, and it's entirely safe and edible. Honeycomb is a collection of hexagonal wax cells built by bees to store honey, pollen, and larvae. It has a unique texture and is often consumed for its flavor, as well as potential health benefits. Here are some aspects of eating honeycomb and its potential health benefits:

1. **Flavor and Texture:**
   - Honeycomb has a pleasant, chewy texture and a delicate, sweet flavor. Eating honeycomb allows you to enjoy both the honey it contains and the waxy comb itself.
2. **Nutrient Content:**
   - Honeycomb contains the same nutrients found in honey, such as natural sugars, vitamins, minerals, and antioxidants. These nutrients can vary depending on the type of flowers the bees visited to collect nectar.
3. **Chewing Wax:**
   - Beeswax is edible, and while it doesn't provide significant nutritional value, it is harmless to chew and swallow in moderate amounts. Some people enjoy chewing honeycomb wax for its unique texture.
4. **Potential Benefits:**
   - The potential health benefits of eating honeycomb are similar to those of consuming honey, as they share many of the same components. These benefits may include:
     - **Antioxidant Properties:** Honeycomb, like honey, contains antioxidants that help neutralize free

radicals in the body, potentially reducing oxidative stress.

- **Anti-Inflammatory Effects:** The antioxidants and other bioactive compounds in honeycomb may contribute to anti-inflammatory effects.
- **Energy Source:** Honeycomb provides a natural source of carbohydrates, primarily in the form of sugars, which can serve as a quick and natural energy source.

5. **Digestibility:**
   - While the wax in honeycomb is digestible, some people prefer not to chew and swallow large amounts of it. Chewing the honeycomb gently and extracting the honey is a common practice.

6. **Local Honey and Allergies:**
   - Some people believe that consuming local honey, including honeycomb, may have potential benefits in managing seasonal allergies. The idea is that exposure to small amounts of local pollen in the honey may help desensitize the immune system. However, scientific evidence supporting this claim is limited.

It's essential to note that individual reactions and preferences may vary, and some people may find the wax texture less appealing. When eating honeycomb, choose high-quality, raw honeycomb from reputable sources to ensure its purity and minimize processing. As with any food, moderation is key, and if you have specific dietary concerns or allergies, it's advisable to consult with a healthcare professional.

What is bee's wax? How do you make it?

Beeswax is a natural substance produced by honeybees (Apis mellifera) through glands on the underside of their abdomen. Bees use beeswax to build honeycomb cells within the hive, where they store honey, pollen, and raise their brood (larvae). The wax is secreted in liquid form by the bees and then hardens into the familiar, waxy structure that forms the comb.

Here's an overview of how beeswax is made by bees:

1. **Secretion of Wax:**
   - Worker bees, which are the female bees, have wax glands on their abdomen. These glands secrete tiny wax droplets.
   - The worker bees chew these wax droplets and mold them into scales on the underside of their abdomen.

2. **Comb Construction:**
   - Worker bees then use these wax scales to build honeycomb cells within the hive. The cells serve various purposes, such as storing honey, pollen, and providing a space for the queen to lay eggs.

3. **Hive Temperature:**
   - The temperature inside the hive plays a crucial role in the process. To keep the wax pliable and workable, the hive temperature needs to be around 91–97 degrees Fahrenheit (33–36 degrees Celsius).

4. **Hardening and Use:**
   - Once the beeswax is molded into the desired shape and the honeycomb structure is complete, it hardens as it cools.
   - The bees use the beeswax comb to store and protect honey, pollen, and the developing brood.

Beekeepers can harvest beeswax when extracting honey from the hive. During honey extraction, the honeycomb is often cut from the frames, and the honey is spun out. The leftover beeswax can then be collected and processed.

To harvest beeswax, the beekeeper typically follows these steps:

1. **Uncapping the Honeycomb:**

- Beekeepers use a hot knife or other tools to uncap the honeycomb, removing a thin layer of wax from the cells to expose the honey inside.

2. **Spinning Honey Extractor:**
   - The frames containing uncapped honeycomb are placed in a honey extractor. The extractor spins the frames rapidly, causing the honey to be flung out of the comb and collected in the extractor's walls.

3. **Separation and Cleaning:**
   - The remaining beeswax, now emptied of honey, is collected. It may still contain some impurities like bee parts and debris.
   - Beekeepers can clean and filter the beeswax to remove these impurities.

4. **Melting and Molding:**
   - The cleaned beeswax can be melted down and molded into various forms. This can include blocks, pellets, or sheets.
   - Beekeepers and artisans use beeswax for various purposes, such as making candles, cosmetics, beeswax wraps, and other products.

Beeswax is valued for its natural properties, including a pleasant honey scent, a golden color, and its ability to burn cleanly in candles. It has been used for centuries in various applications due to its versatility and natural origins.

What is bee's wax good for?

Beeswax is a versatile natural substance that has been used for a wide range of purposes for centuries. Here are some common and beneficial uses of beeswax:

1. **Candle Making:**
   - Beeswax is a popular material for making candles. It burns cleanly, emits a pleasant honey scent, and has a longer burn time compared to some other candle materials.
2. **Cosmetics and Skincare:**
   - Beeswax is a common ingredient in cosmetics and skincare products. It provides a natural emollient, creating a protective barrier on the skin that helps retain moisture. Lip balms, lotions, creams, and salves often contain beeswax.
3. **DIY Skincare Products:**
   - Due to its skin-friendly properties, beeswax is used in homemade skincare products. DIY enthusiasts create natural balms, creams, and ointments using beeswax along with other ingredients like oils and herbs.
4. **Wood and Leather Conditioning:**

- Beeswax can be used to condition and protect wood and leather. It provides a natural, water-resistant coating and enhances the appearance of wooden furniture, cutting boards, and leather goods.

5. **Furniture Polish:**
   - Beeswax-based furniture polish is a natural alternative to commercial furniture polishes. It can be applied to wooden furniture to provide shine and protection.

6. **Waterproofing Fabrics:**
   - Beeswax can be used to waterproof fabrics, making them resistant to water and moisture. This is often done by rubbing or melting beeswax onto outdoor gear, such as jackets and canvas.

7. **Beeswax Wraps:**
   - Beeswax wraps are an eco-friendly alternative to plastic wrap. Cloth is coated with a mixture of beeswax, jojoba oil, and resin, creating a reusable, washable, and moldable wrap for covering food.

8. **Soap Making:**
   - Beeswax is used in soap making to add hardness and texture. It can also contribute to a creamier lather and a longer-lasting bar of soap.

9. **Art and Crafts:**

- Beeswax is a popular medium in art and crafts. Encaustic painting involves using melted beeswax mixed with pigments to create textured and visually striking artwork.

10. **Sealing Envelopes:**
    - Beeswax seals have been historically used to secure and authenticate documents. While less common today, some people use beeswax seals for decorative and nostalgic purposes.

11. **Modeling Wax:**
    - Beeswax can be used as a modeling material in various artistic endeavors, such as sculpture and model-making.

12. **Ear Candles:**
    - Beeswax ear candles, though controversial and not supported by scientific evidence, are sometimes used as a holistic remedy for earwax removal. However, their safety and effectiveness are questioned, and caution is advised.

When using beeswax for any purpose, it's important to choose high-quality, pure beeswax from reputable sources to ensure its natural properties and avoid contaminants. Whether used for practical applications or artistic endeavors, beeswax continues to be valued for its natural and versatile qualities.

How does honey help with heart health? What are some recipes?

Honey may contribute to heart health through several potential mechanisms, primarily related to its natural composition and beneficial compounds. While it's essential to maintain a well-balanced diet and lifestyle for overall cardiovascular health, here are some ways in which honey might positively impact heart health:

1. **Antioxidant Properties:**
    - Honey contains various antioxidants, including polyphenols and flavonoids. Antioxidants help neutralize free radicals in the body, reducing oxidative stress. Chronic oxidative stress is associated with inflammation and cardiovascular diseases.
2. **Anti-Inflammatory Effects:**
    - Some components in honey may exhibit anti-inflammatory properties. Chronic inflammation is linked to the development and progression of heart disease.
3. **Cholesterol Regulation:**
    - There is evidence to suggest that honey may have a positive impact on cholesterol levels. Some studies indicate that honey may help reduce LDL ("bad") cholesterol

levels while increasing HDL ("good") cholesterol levels, contributing to a healthier lipid profile.

4. **Blood Pressure Regulation:**
   - Honey may have a modest impact on blood pressure. Some research suggests that regular consumption of honey might help lower blood pressure, potentially due to its antioxidant and anti-inflammatory effects.

5. **Vasodilation:**
   - Certain compounds in honey may stimulate the production of nitric oxide, a molecule that helps relax and dilate blood vessels. Improved vasodilation can enhance blood flow, contributing to better cardiovascular health.

It's important to note that while honey may have potential cardiovascular benefits, it should be viewed as part of an overall heart-healthy lifestyle. It's not a substitute for a balanced diet, regular physical activity, and other lifestyle factors that contribute to cardiovascular well-being.

Here are a couple of heart-healthy recipes incorporating honey:

1. Honey-Lemon Salmon

Ingredients:

- 4 salmon fillets
- 2 tablespoons honey
- 2 tablespoons soy sauce
- 1 tablespoon Dijon mustard
- 1 tablespoon olive oil
- 1 lemon (juiced)
- Salt and pepper to taste
- Fresh herbs for garnish (parsley, dill)

Instructions:

1. Preheat the oven to 375°F (190°C).
2. In a small bowl, whisk together honey, soy sauce, Dijon mustard, olive oil, lemon juice, salt, and pepper.
3. Place the salmon fillets on a baking sheet lined with parchment paper.
4. Brush the honey mixture over the salmon fillets.
5. Bake in the preheated oven for 12-15 minutes or until the salmon is cooked through.
6. Garnish with fresh herbs before serving.

2. Honey-Yogurt Parfait

Ingredients:

- Greek yogurt
- Fresh berries (strawberries, blueberries, raspberries)
- Granola

- Honey
- Nuts (almonds, walnuts) for crunch (optional)

Instructions:

1. In a glass or bowl, layer Greek yogurt at the bottom.
2. Add a layer of fresh berries.
3. Sprinkle a layer of granola over the berries.
4. Drizzle honey over the granola.
5. Repeat the layers until you reach the top.
6. Top with nuts for added crunch.
7. Enjoy this heart-healthy and delicious parfait!

These recipes incorporate honey into heart-healthy meals, combining its natural sweetness with nutritious ingredients. Remember to choose high-quality, raw honey for maximum potential health benefits. If you have specific health concerns or dietary restrictions, it's advisable to consult with a healthcare professional or a registered dietitian.

How does honey lower cholesterol?

Honey has been suggested to have potential cholesterol-lowering effects, although the mechanisms are not fully understood and more research is needed. Some studies have explored the impact of honey consumption on cholesterol levels, and while the results are promising, it's important to note that individual responses may vary. Here are some potential ways honey may influence cholesterol levels:

1. **Antioxidant Content:**
    - Honey is rich in antioxidants, including polyphenols and flavonoids. Antioxidants help neutralize free radicals in the body, reducing oxidative stress. Oxidative stress is associated with inflammation and damage to cholesterol molecules.
2. **Anti-Inflammatory Properties:**
    - Chronic inflammation is linked to various cardiovascular conditions, including the development and progression of atherosclerosis (hardening and narrowing of the arteries). Some components in honey may have anti-inflammatory effects, which could contribute to heart health.
3. **Effect on LDL Cholesterol:**
    - Several studies have suggested that honey may have a positive impact on low-density lipoprotein (LDL) cholesterol, often referred to as "bad" cholesterol. Elevated LDL cholesterol levels are a risk factor for cardiovascular diseases.

- Honey consumption has been associated with a reduction in LDL cholesterol levels in some individuals.

4. **Increase in HDL Cholesterol:**
   - High-density lipoprotein (HDL) cholesterol is considered "good" cholesterol because it helps remove LDL cholesterol from the bloodstream. Some research suggests that honey consumption may lead to an increase in HDL cholesterol levels, contributing to a healthier lipid profile.

5. **Regulation of Lipid Metabolism:**
   - Honey may influence lipid metabolism, including how the body synthesizes and processes cholesterol. Some studies indicate that honey may have a regulatory effect on enzymes involved in lipid metabolism.

6. **Fiber Content:**
   - While honey is not a significant source of dietary fiber compared to fruits and vegetables, it does contain small amounts. Diets rich in fiber have been associated with improved cholesterol levels.

It's important to approach these potential benefits with some caution and consider the overall context of an individual's diet and lifestyle. Additionally, not all types of honey may have the same effects, as the composition of honey can vary based on factors such as floral source and processing methods.

If you are looking to improve your cholesterol levels, it's crucial to adopt a comprehensive approach that includes a balanced and heart-healthy diet, regular physical activity, and other lifestyle modifications. Before making significant changes to your diet or if you have specific health concerns, it's advisable to consult with a healthcare professional or a registered dietitian for personalized guidance.

How do you use honey to promote burn and wound healing?

Honey has been used for centuries as a natural remedy for wound healing and burns. Its antimicrobial, anti-inflammatory, and wound-healing properties make it a beneficial option for promoting the recovery of minor burns and wounds. Here's how you can use honey for this purpose:

For Minor Wounds:

1. **Clean the Wound:**
   - Before applying honey, ensure that the wound is clean. Wash the affected area gently with mild soap and water.
2. **Apply Honey:**

- Use a clean, sterile applicator or cotton swab to apply a thin layer of honey directly to the wound. Ensure that the honey covers the entire wound.

3. **Cover the Wound (Optional):**
   - Depending on the location of the wound, you may choose to cover it with a sterile bandage or gauze to protect it from external contaminants.

4. **Reapply as Needed:**
   - Reapply honey and change the dressing regularly, at least once or twice a day. Honey's antimicrobial properties can help prevent infection and support the natural healing process.

For Minor Burns:

1. **Cool the Burn:**
   - For minor burns, cool the affected area with cold running water for about 10-20 minutes. Avoid using ice directly on the burn.

2. **Gently Pat Dry:**
   - Gently pat the burn area dry with a clean, soft cloth or towel.

3. **Apply Honey:**
   - Once the burn is dry, apply a thin layer of honey directly to the burn. Honey's natural

properties can help soothe the burn and support healing.

4. **Cover with a Non-Stick Dressing (Optional):**
   - You may choose to cover the burn with a non-stick dressing or gauze. This can help protect the burn while allowing the honey to work.

5. **Reapply as Needed:**
   - Reapply honey and change the dressing regularly, at least once or twice a day. Monitor the burn for signs of infection, such as increased redness, swelling, or pus.

Tips and Considerations:

- Use raw, unprocessed honey for its optimal healing properties. Processing can reduce the honey's effectiveness.
- Manuka honey, derived from the nectar of the Manuka tree, is known for its potent antimicrobial properties and is often used for wound healing.
- If you have allergies to bee products, it's essential to perform a patch test or consult with a healthcare professional before using honey topically.
- In case of severe burns or wounds, or if signs of infection persist, seek medical attention promptly.

While honey can be beneficial for minor wounds and burns, it's crucial to note that serious injuries require professional medical attention. Always consult with a healthcare professional for appropriate guidance, especially for more severe burns or wounds that may need specialized care.

If you are allergic to bees, can you use honey? Can consuming honey reverse the reaction to bee allergies?

If you have a known allergy to bees, it's crucial to exercise caution and seek advice from a healthcare professional before using or consuming honey. While the risk of an allergic reaction to honey is generally low, there is a potential for cross-contamination with bee-related allergens. Bee-related allergens may be present in trace amounts in honey due to pollen or other bee particles.

Here are some important considerations:

1. **Consultation with Healthcare Professional:**
    - Individuals with a known allergy to bees should consult with an allergist or healthcare professional before incorporating honey into their diet or using it topically.
2. **Risk of Cross-Contamination:**
    - Honey can contain small amounts of bee-related allergens, such as pollen or bee

particles. While the concentration is usually minimal, it can pose a risk to individuals with severe bee allergies.

3. **Potential for Sensitization:**
   - Consuming honey is not known to reverse or eliminate bee allergies. In fact, individuals with a known bee allergy should avoid exposure to bee products to prevent sensitization or the potential for more severe allergic reactions.

4. **Allergenic Proteins:**
   - Allergenic proteins from bees, such as venom proteins, are not typically found in honey in significant amounts. However, the presence of trace amounts is possible, and the risk should be assessed based on the individual's specific allergy profile.

5. **Pollen Allergies:**
   - Some individuals may be allergic to pollen and experience symptoms such as hay fever. Honey contains pollen, and in rare cases, it may trigger allergic reactions in individuals with pollen allergies.

It's essential to differentiate between bee venom allergies (resulting from stings) and allergies related to bee products like honey. While reactions to honey are rare, individuals with a history of severe allergic reactions, anaphylaxis, or bee venom allergies should take precautions.

If you suspect an allergy or experience symptoms such as itching, swelling, difficulty breathing, or hives after consuming honey, seek immediate medical attention. An allergist can conduct specific tests to assess the risk of allergic reactions and provide personalized recommendations.

In summary, if you have a known bee allergy, consult with a healthcare professional before using honey or any bee-related products. They can assess your specific situation, conduct allergy testing if needed, and provide guidance on safe practices to avoid potential allergic reactions.

What are the secret benefits of honey?

Honey is renowned for its natural sweetness, but it also offers a range of potential health benefits and practical uses beyond just being a delicious sweetener. Here are some "secret" benefits of honey:

1. **Antioxidant Power:**
   - Honey is rich in antioxidants, including polyphenols and flavonoids. Antioxidants help combat oxidative stress, supporting

overall health and potentially reducing the risk of chronic diseases.

2. **Cough and Throat Soothing:**
   - Honey is a common home remedy for soothing a sore throat and relieving coughs. Its natural sweetness can help coat the throat, while its antimicrobial properties may provide additional benefits.

3. **Wound Healing:**
   - Honey has been used for centuries to aid in wound healing. Its antimicrobial and anti-inflammatory properties can help prevent infection and support the natural healing process for minor cuts and burns.

4. **Digestive Health:**
   - Consuming honey in moderation may have positive effects on digestive health. It has prebiotic properties that can promote the growth of beneficial bacteria in the gut, contributing to a healthy digestive system.

5. **Natural Energy Source:**
   - Honey is a natural source of carbohydrates, primarily in the form of glucose and fructose. This makes it a quick and easily digestible energy source, making it a popular choice for athletes or those needing a natural energy boost.

6. **Improved Sleep:**

- Honey may contribute to better sleep when consumed with warm milk or herbal tea before bedtime. It is thought to promote the release of serotonin, which converts to melatonin, a hormone that regulates sleep.

7. **Skin Care:**
   - Honey's moisturizing and antibacterial properties make it a popular ingredient in skincare products. It can be used in face masks, cleansers, and moisturizers to promote healthy skin.

8. **Allergy Symptom Relief:**
   - Some people believe that consuming local honey may help alleviate seasonal allergy symptoms. The idea is that exposure to small amounts of local pollen in honey may desensitize the immune system. However, scientific evidence supporting this claim is limited.

9. **Improved Memory:**
   - There is some preliminary research suggesting that honey may have cognitive benefits. A study found that honey consumption was associated with better spatial memory in postmenopausal women.

10. **Hangover Relief:**
    - Honey may help alleviate hangover symptoms. Consuming honey on toast or with warm water can provide a source of

easily digestible sugars to help restore depleted glycogen levels after alcohol consumption.

11. **Dandruff Treatment:**

   - Honey can be used in homemade hair masks to address dandruff. Its antibacterial and moisturizing properties may help soothe the scalp and reduce flakiness.

12. **Natural Preservative:**

   - Honey's low water content and acidic pH make it an inhospitable environment for bacteria and microorganisms. It has been used historically as a natural preservative for foods.

While honey offers these potential benefits, it's important to consume it in moderation due to its calorie and sugar content. Additionally, individual responses to honey can vary, and specific health conditions may warrant caution or avoidance. Always consult with a healthcare professional for personalized advice based on your health status and individual needs.

What are 20 recipes including honey for beneficial reasons? What are they good for?

Here are 20 recipes that include honey for various beneficial reasons, covering a range of purposes such as immune support, energy, skincare, and more. Remember to use high-quality, raw honey to maximize potential health benefits. Additionally, individual responses to these recipes may vary, and if you have specific health concerns or allergies, it's advisable to consult with a healthcare professional.

1. Honey-Lemon Tea:

- **Benefit:** Soothing for sore throats, provides vitamin C.
- **Recipe:** Mix hot water, lemon juice, and honey. Drink as a comforting tea.

2. Honey and Cinnamon Oatmeal:

- **Benefit:** Balanced breakfast for sustained energy.
- **Recipe:** Stir honey and cinnamon into your morning oatmeal.

3. Honey Mustard Dressing:

- **Benefit:** Healthier alternative to store-bought dressings.
- **Recipe:** Combine honey, Dijon mustard, olive oil, and vinegar for a tasty salad dressing.

4. Turmeric Honey Golden Milk:

- **Benefit:** Anti-inflammatory and immune support.

- **Recipe:** Mix turmeric, honey, and warm milk for a soothing golden milk.

5. Honey-Glazed Salmon:

- **Benefit:** Omega-3 fatty acids for heart health.
- **Recipe:** Brush salmon fillets with a mixture of honey, soy sauce, and garlic before baking.

6. Honey Yogurt Parfait:

- **Benefit:** Probiotics for gut health.
- **Recipe:** Layer Greek yogurt with honey, granola, and fresh berries.

7. Honey Garlic Chicken Stir-Fry:

- **Benefit:** Protein-packed and flavorful.
- **Recipe:** Stir-fry chicken, vegetables, and a honey-garlic sauce.

8. Honey Citrus Salad:

- **Benefit:** Vitamin-rich, hydrating salad.
- **Recipe:** Toss mixed greens, citrus segments, and a honey-lime vinaigrette.

9. Honey Almond Energy Bites:

- **Benefit:** Quick energy boost, great for snacking.

- **Recipe:** Mix rolled oats, almond butter, honey, and chopped nuts. Form into bite-sized balls.

These recipes showcase the versatility of honey in both sweet and savory dishes, as well as in skincare routines. Experiment with these ideas to enjoy the potential health benefits and delicious flavors that honey can offer.

How do you make honey ginger lemonade? What is the benefit of Honey Ginger Lemonade?

Honey ginger lemonade is not only a refreshing and flavorful beverage but also offers potential health benefits. The combination of honey, ginger, and lemon provides a delicious blend of sweetness, warmth, and citrusy goodness. Here's a simple recipe for making honey ginger lemonade:

Honey Ginger Lemonade Recipe:

Ingredients:

- 4 cups water
- 1/2 cup fresh lemon juice (about 4 lemons)
- 1/4 cup honey (adjust to taste)
- 1-2 tablespoons fresh ginger, grated
- Ice cubes
- Lemon slices and fresh mint for garnish (optional)

Instructions:

1. **Prepare the Ginger:**
   - Peel and grate the fresh ginger. You can adjust the quantity based on your preference for ginger flavor.
2. **Make the Honey Ginger Syrup:**
   - In a small saucepan, combine the grated ginger, honey, and 1 cup of water.
   - Bring the mixture to a simmer over medium heat, stirring until the honey dissolves.
   - Let it simmer for 5-7 minutes to infuse the ginger flavor into the syrup.
   - Remove from heat and allow it to cool. Strain the syrup to remove the ginger pieces.
3. **Mix the Lemonade:**
   - In a large pitcher, combine the fresh lemon juice, honey ginger syrup, and the remaining 3 cups of water.
   - Stir well to ensure the ingredients are thoroughly mixed.
4. **Chill and Serve:**
   - Refrigerate the lemonade for at least 1-2 hours to chill.
   - Serve over ice and garnish with lemon slices and fresh mint if desired.
5. **Adjust Sweetness:**

- Taste the lemonade and adjust the sweetness by adding more honey if needed.

Enjoy your homemade honey ginger lemonade!

Benefits of Honey Ginger Lemonade:

1. **Immune Support:**
   - Ginger and lemon are known for their immune-boosting properties. They contain antioxidants and vitamins that may help support the immune system.
2. **Digestive Aid:**
   - Ginger has long been used to aid digestion. It may help alleviate nausea, indigestion, and bloating.
3. **Anti-Inflammatory Effects:**
   - Both ginger and honey have anti-inflammatory properties that may help reduce inflammation in the body.
4. **Sore Throat Relief:**
   - Honey and lemon are commonly used for soothing sore throats. The honey provides a coating effect, while lemon offers vitamin C.
5. **Hydration:**

- Staying hydrated is essential for overall health. Lemonade can be a tasty way to increase fluid intake.

6. **Refreshing Flavor:**
   - The combination of honey, ginger, and lemon creates a deliciously refreshing flavor that can be enjoyed on a hot day or as a pick-me-up.

Remember that individual responses to ingredients may vary, and if you have specific health concerns or allergies, it's advisable to consult with a healthcare professional. Additionally, moderation is key when consuming honey, especially if you are watching your sugar intake.

What is the benefit of a honey turmeric face mask? What is the recipe?

A honey turmeric face mask is a popular natural skincare remedy that may offer various benefits for the skin. Both honey and turmeric are known for their potential skincare properties, including anti-inflammatory, antioxidant, and moisturizing effects. Here are some potential benefits and a simple recipe for a honey turmeric face mask:

Benefits of a Honey Turmeric Face Mask:

1. **Anti-Inflammatory Properties:**
   - Turmeric contains curcumin, a compound known for its anti-inflammatory properties. This can help soothe irritated skin and reduce redness.
2. **Antioxidant Boost:**
   - Both honey and turmeric are rich in antioxidants that can help neutralize free radicals, contributing to a healthier complexion.
3. **Moisturizing and Hydrating:**
   - Honey is a natural humectant, meaning it helps retain moisture. This, combined with turmeric, can provide hydration to the skin.
4. **Brightening Effect:**
   - Turmeric is believed to have skin-brightening properties, which may help improve the appearance of dark spots and uneven skin tone.
5. **Acne Management:**
   - The antibacterial properties of honey and the anti-inflammatory properties of turmeric may help manage acne and promote clearer skin.

Honey Turmeric Face Mask Recipe:

Ingredients:

- 1 tablespoon turmeric powder

- 1 tablespoon raw honey

Instructions:

1. **Mixing:**
   - In a small bowl, combine the turmeric powder and raw honey. Mix well until you have a smooth, consistent paste.
2. **Application:**
   - Before applying the mask, cleanse your face to remove any makeup or impurities.
   - Using clean fingers or a brush, apply an even layer of the honey turmeric paste to your face, avoiding the eye area.
3. **Relaxing Time:**
   - Allow the mask to sit on your face for about 15–20 minutes. You may experience a slight tingling sensation, which is normal.
4. **Rinsing:**
   - After the designated time, gently rinse off the mask with warm water. You may want to use a soft washcloth to help remove the yellow tint from turmeric.
5. **Moisturize:**
   - Follow up with your regular moisturizer to lock in hydration.

Important Tips:

- **Patch Test:**

- Perform a patch test before applying the mask to your entire face to ensure you don't have an adverse reaction.
- **Turmeric Stains:**
    - Turmeric has a yellow pigment that can temporarily stain the skin. If you notice some staining, it should fade after additional cleansing.
- **Frequency:**
    - Use the mask 1–2 times per week to avoid overexfoliation and potential skin sensitivity.
- **Cautions:**
    - Avoid this mask if you have an allergy to honey or turmeric. If you have sensitive skin, consult with a dermatologist before trying new skincare ingredients.

This honey turmeric face mask can be a natural addition to your skincare routine, offering potential benefits for a radiant and healthy complexion. However, individual skin reactions may vary, so discontinue use if you experience any irritation and consult with a dermatologist if you have specific skin concerns.

How do you make cucumber mint honey water? What are the benefits?

Cucumber mint honey water is a refreshing and hydrating beverage that combines the mild flavor of cucumber with the cooling effect of mint and the sweetness of honey. It's a delightful way to stay hydrated, especially on hot days. Here's a simple recipe for making cucumber mint honey water along with some potential benefits:

Cucumber Mint Honey Water Recipe:

Ingredients:

- 1 medium cucumber, washed and thinly sliced
- A handful of fresh mint leaves, washed
- 1-2 tablespoons honey (adjust to taste)
- 4 cups cold water
- Ice cubes (optional)
- Lemon slices for garnish (optional)

Instructions:

1. **Prepare the Cucumber and Mint:**
   - Wash the cucumber and mint leaves thoroughly. Slice the cucumber into thin rounds.
2. **Assemble in a Pitcher:**
   - In a large pitcher, combine the cucumber slices and fresh mint leaves.
3. **Add Honey:**

- Drizzle honey over the cucumber and mint. Adjust the amount of honey based on your sweetness preference.

4. **Muddle (Optional):**
   - Using a muddler or the back of a spoon, gently press down on the cucumber slices and mint leaves to release their flavors. This step is optional but can enhance the infusion.

5. **Add Water:**
   - Pour cold water into the pitcher, covering the cucumber and mint.

6. **Stir Well:**
   - Stir the mixture well to combine the ingredients.

7. **Chill:**
   - Place the pitcher in the refrigerator to chill for at least 1-2 hours. This allows the flavors to infuse into the water.

8. **Serve:**
   - Pour the cucumber mint honey water into glasses over ice cubes if desired. Garnish with lemon slices for an extra burst of freshness.

9. **Enjoy:**
   - Sip and enjoy the refreshing and hydrating flavors of cucumber, mint, and honey.

Benefits of Cucumber Mint Honey Water:

1. **Hydration:**
   - Cucumber is made up of over 95% water, making this infused water an excellent hydrating beverage.
2. **Antioxidant Properties:**
   - Mint and cucumber both contain antioxidants that help combat free radicals in the body, contributing to overall health.
3. **Digestive Support:**
   - Cucumber is known for its digestive benefits, and mint may help soothe an upset stomach. This combination can provide gentle digestive support.
4. **Mood Booster:**
   - The refreshing and invigorating aroma of mint is known to have mood-boosting effects, promoting a sense of alertness and well-being.
5. **Low-Calorie Alternative:**
   - Cucumber mint honey water is a low-calorie alternative to sugary beverages, making it a healthier choice for those looking to reduce calorie intake.
6. **Natural Sweetness:**
   - The addition of honey provides natural sweetness without the need for refined sugars, making it a better option for those watching their sugar intake.
7. **Vitamin C:**

- Cucumber and mint contribute small amounts of vitamin C, which supports the immune system and promotes healthy skin.

Remember to customize the recipe to suit your taste preferences, and feel free to experiment with other herbs or fruits for additional flavors. This beverage is not only enjoyable but also a nutritious and hydrating addition to your daily routine.

What is the recipe for honey sesame roasted vegetables?

Honey sesame roasted vegetables are a delicious and nutritious side dish that combines the natural sweetness of honey with the nutty flavor of sesame seeds. This recipe is versatile, allowing you to use a variety of vegetables based on your preferences. Here's a basic recipe for honey sesame roasted vegetables:

Honey Sesame Roasted Vegetables Recipe:

Ingredients:

- 4 cups mixed vegetables, chopped into bite-sized pieces (e.g., carrots, broccoli, bell peppers, zucchini, cauliflower)

- 2 tablespoons olive oil
- 2 tablespoons honey
- 1 tablespoon soy sauce (or tamari for a gluten-free option)
- 1 tablespoon sesame oil
- 2 tablespoons sesame seeds
- Salt and pepper to taste
- Optional: Garlic powder, ginger powder, or red pepper flakes for added flavor

Instructions:

1. **Preheat the Oven:**
   - Preheat your oven to 400°F (200°C).
2. **Prepare the Vegetables:**
   - Wash and chop the vegetables into bite-sized pieces. Ensure they are similar in size for even roasting.
3. **Prepare the Honey Sesame Glaze:**
   - In a small bowl, whisk together olive oil, honey, soy sauce, sesame oil, and any optional seasonings (garlic powder, ginger powder, red pepper flakes).
4. **Coat the Vegetables:**
   - Place the chopped vegetables in a large mixing bowl. Pour the honey sesame glaze over the vegetables and toss until the vegetables are evenly coated.
5. **Arrange on a Baking Sheet:**

- Spread the coated vegetables in a single layer on a baking sheet lined with parchment paper or lightly greased.

6. **Roast in the Oven:**
   - Roast in the preheated oven for 20-25 minutes or until the vegetables are tender and slightly caramelized. Stir the vegetables halfway through the roasting time for even cooking.

7. **Add Sesame Seeds:**
   - Sprinkle sesame seeds over the roasted vegetables during the last 5 minutes of cooking. This adds a crunchy texture and enhances the sesame flavor.

8. **Season and Serve:**
   - Remove the baking sheet from the oven. Season the roasted vegetables with salt and pepper to taste. Toss gently to combine.

9. **Garnish (Optional):**
   - Garnish with additional sesame seeds and chopped fresh herbs like parsley or cilantro if desired.

10. **Serve Warm:**
    - Serve the honey sesame roasted vegetables warm as a side dish or over a bed of cooked quinoa or rice for a complete meal.

Tips and Variations:

- Customize the vegetable selection based on your preferences or what's in season.
- Experiment with additional seasonings such as crushed red pepper flakes for a bit of heat or a squeeze of fresh lemon juice for brightness.
- Consider adding protein sources like tofu, chicken, or shrimp to make it a well-rounded meal.

This recipe offers a delightful combination of sweet and savory flavors, making it a perfect side dish for a variety of meals. Adjust the ingredients and quantities to suit your taste preferences and dietary requirements.

What are the benefits to a honey and lavender infused oil? How do you make it? How do you use the oil?

Honey and lavender-infused oil is a versatile natural product that combines the soothing properties of lavender with the moisturizing qualities of honey. This infused oil can be used for various purposes, including skincare and aromatherapy. Here are the potential benefits, a simple recipe for making honey and lavender-infused oil, and ways to use it:

Benefits of Honey and Lavender Infused Oil:

1. **Calming and Relaxing:**
   - Lavender is known for its calming and stress-relieving properties. Using the infused oil in aromatherapy or massage may promote relaxation.
2. **Moisturizing:**
   - Honey is a natural humectant, helping the skin retain moisture. The infused oil can be used to moisturize dry or irritated skin.
3. **Antioxidant Properties:**
   - Both honey and lavender contain antioxidants that may help protect the skin from free radicals, supporting overall skin health.
4. **Soothing for Irritated Skin:**
   - Lavender is known for its soothing properties, which can be beneficial for irritated or sensitive skin.
5. **Aromatherapy:**
   - The pleasant aroma of lavender can have therapeutic effects, promoting a sense of calm and well-being.

Honey and Lavender Infused Oil Recipe:

Ingredients:

- 1 cup carrier oil (such as sweet almond oil, jojoba oil, or olive oil)
- 1/4 cup dried lavender flowers
- 2 tablespoons raw honey

Instructions:

1. **Prepare the Lavender Flowers:**
   - Ensure the lavender flowers are clean and free of debris. If needed, gently shake or tap them to remove any loose particles.
2. **Combine Ingredients:**
   - In a clean, dry glass jar, combine the dried lavender flowers and honey.
3. **Heat the Carrier Oil:**
   - In a small saucepan, heat the carrier oil over low heat until it is warm but not boiling. This helps the oil better absorb the properties of the lavender and honey.
4. **Infuse the Oil:**
   - Pour the warm carrier oil over the lavender flowers and honey in the jar. Stir gently to ensure the honey dissolves.
5. **Seal and Steep:**
   - Seal the jar tightly and place it in a cool, dark place to steep for about 2-4 weeks. Shake the jar occasionally to help the ingredients infuse.
6. **Strain the Oil:**

- After the steeping period, strain the oil using a fine mesh strainer or cheesecloth to remove the lavender flowers and any sediment.

7. **Store the Infused Oil:**
   - Transfer the strained oil into a clean, airtight glass container. Store it in a cool, dark place.

How to Use Honey and Lavender Infused Oil:

1. **Massage Oil:**
   - Warm the infused oil slightly and use it as a massage oil to promote relaxation and soothe the skin.
2. **Moisturizer:**
   - Apply a small amount of the infused oil to dry or irritated skin areas as a moisturizer.
3. **Aromatherapy:**
   - Add a few drops of the infused oil to a diffuser for a calming and fragrant atmosphere.
4. **Bath Oil:**
   - Add a few drops of the infused oil to your bathwater for a luxurious and relaxing experience.
5. **Hair Treatment:**

- Apply a small amount of the infused oil to the ends of your hair as a conditioning treatment.
6. **Homemade Salves or Balms:**
   - Use the infused oil as a base for homemade salves or balms for skin soothing and moisturizing.

Remember to perform a patch test before applying the infused oil to a larger area of the skin to ensure you do not have an adverse reaction. If you experience any irritation, discontinue use. This homemade infused oil can be a delightful addition to your natural skincare and wellness routine.

What are the benefits of honey walnut banana bread? How do you make it?

Honey walnut banana bread is a delightful twist on the classic banana bread, incorporating the rich flavor of honey and the crunchy texture of walnuts. This combination not only enhances the taste but also brings potential health benefits from the natural ingredients. Here are some benefits and a simple recipe for making honey walnut banana bread:

Benefits of Honey Walnut Banana Bread:

1. **Natural Sweetener:**

- Honey serves as a natural sweetener, providing a sweet taste without the need for refined sugars.

2. **Nutrient-Rich:**
   - Walnuts are a good source of omega-3 fatty acids, antioxidants, and essential nutrients like vitamin E.

3. **Moisture and Flavor:**
   - Honey contributes moisture to the bread, resulting in a soft and tender texture. It also adds a distinctive flavor that complements the bananas.

4. **Antioxidant Properties:**
   - Both honey and walnuts contain antioxidants that can help neutralize free radicals in the body.

5. **Protein and Healthy Fats:**
   - Walnuts are a source of protein and healthy fats, providing a satisfying and nourishing element to the banana bread.

Honey Walnut Banana Bread Recipe:

Ingredients:

- 3 ripe bananas, mashed
- 1/3 cup melted butter or coconut oil
- 1/2 cup honey
- 1 teaspoon vanilla extract
- 1 teaspoon baking soda

- 1/4 teaspoon salt
- 1 3/4 cups all-purpose flour
- 1/2 cup chopped walnuts
- Optional: Additional walnuts for topping

Instructions:

1. **Preheat the Oven:**
   - Preheat your oven to 350°F (175°C). Grease a 9x5-inch (23x13 cm) loaf pan.
2. **Mash the Bananas:**
   - In a large mixing bowl, mash the ripe bananas with a fork or potato masher until smooth.
3. **Add Wet Ingredients:**
   - Add the melted butter or coconut oil, honey, and vanilla extract to the mashed bananas. Mix well to combine.
4. **Combine Dry Ingredients:**
   - In a separate bowl, whisk together the flour, baking soda, and salt.
5. **Combine Wet and Dry Ingredients:**
   - Gradually add the dry ingredients to the banana mixture, stirring until just combined. Be careful not to overmix.
6. **Fold in Walnuts:**
   - Gently fold in the chopped walnuts into the batter.
7. **Pour into Loaf Pan:**

- Pour the batter into the greased loaf pan. If desired, sprinkle additional walnuts on top for decoration.

8. **Bake:**
   - Bake in the preheated oven for 60-70 minutes or until a toothpick inserted into the center comes out clean or with a few moist crumbs.

9. **Cool and Slice:**
   - Allow the banana bread to cool in the pan for about 10 minutes, then transfer it to a wire rack to cool completely before slicing.

10. **Enjoy:**
    - Slice and enjoy your honey walnut banana bread with a cup of tea or coffee!

Tips:

- **Ripe Bananas:** Use ripe bananas for the best flavor. The riper, the better, as they add natural sweetness.
- **Honey:** Choose high-quality, raw honey for its optimal flavor and potential health benefits.
- **Storage:** Store the banana bread in an airtight container at room temperature for a day or two. For longer storage, refrigerate or freeze slices.

This honey walnut banana bread is a delicious and wholesome treat that can be enjoyed as a snack, breakfast, or dessert. Feel free to customize it by adding other ingredients like chocolate chips, dried fruit, or spices to suit your taste preferences.

How do you make Honey chamomile popsicles? Why are they good for you?

Honey chamomile popsicles are not only a refreshing treat but also potentially offer some health benefits. Chamomile is known for its calming properties, and when combined with honey, it creates a delightful and soothing popsicle. Here's a simple recipe for making honey chamomile popsicles and some reasons they may be considered good for you:

Honey Chamomile Popsicles Recipe:

Ingredients:

- 2 chamomile tea bags or 2 tablespoons dried chamomile flowers
- 1 1/2 cups boiling water
- 2 tablespoons honey (adjust to taste)
- 1 tablespoon lemon juice (optional, for a hint of citrus)
- Popsicle molds and sticks

Instructions:

1. **Brew Chamomile Tea:**
   - Steep the chamomile tea bags or dried chamomile flowers in boiling water for about 5-7 minutes. This creates a chamomile-infused tea.
2. **Sweeten with Honey:**
   - While the tea is still warm, add honey to the chamomile infusion. Stir well until the honey is fully dissolved. Adjust the sweetness to your liking.
3. **Optional: Add Lemon Juice:**
   - If desired, add lemon juice to the chamomile-honey mixture for a touch of citrus flavor. Stir to combine.
4. **Cool the Mixture:**
   - Allow the chamomile-honey mixture to cool to room temperature.
5. **Pour into Popsicle Molds:**
   - Once cooled, pour the chamomile-honey mixture into popsicle molds. Leave a little space at the top for the mixture to expand as it freezes.
6. **Insert Popsicle Sticks:**
   - Place popsicle sticks into each mold, making sure they are centered.
7. **Freeze:**
   - Freeze the popsicles for at least 4-6 hours or until completely frozen.
8. **Unmold and Enjoy:**

- Once frozen, run the popsicle mold under warm water for a few seconds to loosen the popsicles. Gently pull them out and enjoy!

Why Honey Chamomile Popsicles May Be Good for You:

1. **Calming and Relaxing:**
    - Chamomile is renowned for its calming and relaxing properties. Consuming chamomile in popsicle form may be a pleasant way to enjoy its soothing effects.
2. **Digestive Support:**
    - Chamomile has been traditionally used to aid digestion and relieve digestive discomfort. Enjoying chamomile-infused popsicles may contribute to digestive well-being.
3. **Antioxidant Properties:**
    - Both chamomile and honey contain antioxidants that help combat oxidative stress in the body.
4. **Throat Soothing:**
    - Honey is known for its throat-soothing properties. Combining honey with chamomile in popsicle form may provide a gentle and enjoyable way to soothe the throat.
5. **Hydration:**

- Popsicles are a hydrating treat, and the chamomile tea base ensures you get additional fluid intake.

6. **Natural Sweetener:**
   - Honey serves as a natural sweetener, providing sweetness without the need for refined sugars.

7. **Caffeine-Free:**
   - Chamomile is caffeine-free, making these popsicles a suitable option for relaxation any time of day.

8. **Flavorful and Refreshing:**
   - The combination of chamomile, honey, and optional lemon juice creates a flavorful and refreshing popsicle that can be enjoyed during warm weather.

It's important to note that individual responses to chamomile may vary. If you have allergies or concerns, consult with a healthcare professional before regularly consuming chamomile products. Additionally, moderation is key when consuming honey, especially for individuals watching their sugar intake.

What is a honey ginger shot for immunity shots? What is the recipe?

A honey ginger shot for immunity is a concentrated beverage that combines the immune-boosting properties of ginger and honey. This potent shot is often consumed in small quantities and is believed to have various health benefits, including supporting the immune system and providing a burst of energy. Here's a simple recipe for making a honey ginger immunity shot:

Honey Ginger Immunity Shot Recipe:

Ingredients:

- 1 tablespoon fresh ginger, peeled and grated
- 1 tablespoon raw honey
- 1/2 lemon, juiced
- 1/4 teaspoon turmeric powder (optional)
- Pinch of cayenne pepper (optional)
- 1/2 cup warm water

Instructions:

1. **Prepare the Ginger:**
   - Peel and grate a tablespoon of fresh ginger. You can adjust the quantity based on your tolerance for the ginger's spiciness.
2. **Juice the Lemon:**
   - Squeeze the juice from half a lemon to get about 1 tablespoon of fresh lemon juice.
3. **Mix the Ingredients:**
   - In a small bowl or cup, combine the grated ginger, raw honey, lemon juice, turmeric

powder (if using), and a pinch of cayenne pepper (if you like it spicy).

4. **Add Warm Water:**
   - Pour 1/2 cup of warm water into the mixture. Warm water helps dissolve the honey and enhances the overall soothing effect.
5. **Stir Well:**
   - Stir the ingredients well until the honey is completely dissolved and the mixture is well combined.
6. **Strain (Optional):**
   - If you prefer a smoother shot, you can strain the mixture using a fine mesh strainer or cheesecloth to remove the ginger pulp.
7. **Pour into Shot Glasses:**
   - Pour the honey ginger immunity shot into small shot glasses.
8. **Consume:**
   - Consume the shot in one go. Be prepared for the spiciness of ginger, which can provide a warming sensation.

Additional Tips:

- **Adjust Spice Levels:**
  - You can adjust the spiciness of the shot by varying the amount of ginger and cayenne

pepper. Start with smaller amounts if you are sensitive to spice.

- **Turmeric Option:**
  - Turmeric is known for its anti-inflammatory properties. Adding turmeric powder to the shot can provide additional health benefits.
- **Fresh Ingredients:**
  - Use fresh ginger and real honey for optimal flavor and potential health benefits. Avoid using processed honey, as raw honey contains more beneficial compounds.
- **Consistency:**
  - Consuming a honey ginger shot regularly is a common practice, especially during the colder months, to help support the immune system. However, it's essential to consult with a healthcare professional if you have specific health concerns.

This honey ginger immunity shot is a quick and potent way to incorporate immune-boosting ingredients into your routine. Keep in mind that individual responses to these ingredients may vary, and it's advisable to start with smaller amounts, especially if you are new to consuming ginger shots.

How do you make a honey avocado face mask? What is the recipe?

A honey avocado face mask is a simple yet luxurious way to nourish and hydrate your skin. Avocado is rich in healthy fats, vitamins, and antioxidants, while honey provides moisture and has antibacterial properties. Here's a basic recipe for a honey avocado face mask:

Honey Avocado Face Mask Recipe:

Ingredients:

- 1/2 ripe avocado
- 2 tablespoons raw honey

Instructions:

1. **Prepare the Avocado:**
   - Scoop out the flesh of half a ripe avocado and place it in a bowl. Make sure the avocado is ripe, as it will be easier to mash and apply to your face.
2. **Mash the Avocado:**
   - Mash the avocado using a fork or spoon until you achieve a smooth consistency. Ensure there are no lumps.
3. **Add Honey:**
   - Add 2 tablespoons of raw honey to the mashed avocado. You can adjust the quantity of honey based on your

preference and the desired consistency of the mask.

4. **Mix Well:**
   - Mix the avocado and honey thoroughly until you have a smooth and well-blended mixture.

5. **Application:**
   - Cleanse your face before applying the mask. Using clean fingers or a brush, apply the honey avocado mixture evenly to your face, avoiding the eye area.

6. **Relax:**
   - Once the mask is applied, relax and let it sit on your face for about 15-20 minutes. You can use this time to unwind, read a book, or simply enjoy a moment of self-care.

7. **Rinse Off:**
   - After the designated time, gently rinse the mask off with lukewarm water. Pat your face dry with a clean towel.

8. **Moisturize:**
   - Follow up with your regular moisturizer to lock in the hydration from the mask.

Optional Additions:

- **Lemon Juice:**
  - For a brightening effect, you can add a teaspoon of fresh lemon juice to the mask.

Lemon juice contains natural acids that may help exfoliate the skin gently.

- **Yogurt:**
  - A tablespoon of plain yogurt can be added for its probiotic benefits and lactic acid content, which may contribute to a smoother complexion.
- **Oatmeal:**
  - For additional exfoliation, consider incorporating finely ground oatmeal into the mask. This can help slough off dead skin cells.

Benefits of a Honey Avocado Face Mask:

1. **Hydration:**
   - Avocado is rich in healthy fats that can moisturize and nourish the skin. Honey adds an extra layer of hydration.
2. **Antioxidant Boost:**
   - Both avocado and honey contain antioxidants that help protect the skin from free radicals.
3. **Soothing and Calming:**
   - The combination of honey and avocado can have a soothing and calming effect on the skin, making it beneficial for sensitive or irritated skin.
4. **Vitamins and Nutrients:**

- Avocado is a good source of vitamins E and C, which can contribute to healthier-looking skin.

5. **Gentle Exfoliation (with Optional Additions):**
   - Lemon juice and yogurt can provide gentle exfoliation, promoting a smoother complexion.

Remember to perform a patch test before applying the mask to your entire face, especially if you have sensitive skin or are allergic to any of the ingredients. Enjoy the pampering and nourishing benefits of this honey avocado face mask as part of your skincare routine.

What are the benefits to spiced honey hot chocolate? What is the recipe?

Spiced honey hot chocolate is a delightful and comforting beverage that combines the richness of hot chocolate with the warmth of spices and the sweetness of honey. This flavorful drink not only satisfies your chocolate cravings but also offers additional layers of taste and potential health benefits. Here's a simple recipe for spiced honey hot chocolate and some reasons why it might be considered beneficial:

Spiced Honey Hot Chocolate Recipe:

Ingredients:

- 2 cups milk (dairy or non-dairy alternatives like almond, soy, or oat milk)
- 2 tablespoons unsweetened cocoa powder
- 2-3 tablespoons honey (adjust to taste)
- 1/2 teaspoon ground cinnamon
- 1/4 teaspoon ground nutmeg
- 1/4 teaspoon vanilla extract
- A pinch of cayenne pepper (optional, for a hint of heat)
- Whipped cream and additional cinnamon for garnish (optional)

Instructions:

1. **Prepare the Hot Chocolate Base:**
   - In a small saucepan, heat the milk over medium heat until it's warm but not boiling.
2. **Add Cocoa Powder:**
   - Whisk in the cocoa powder until it's fully dissolved and the milk is well combined.
3. **Sweeten with Honey:**
   - Add honey to the hot chocolate base, adjusting the amount based on your sweetness preference. Stir until the honey is fully dissolved.
4. **Add Spices:**
   - Mix in the ground cinnamon, ground nutmeg, vanilla extract, and cayenne

pepper (if using). Continue to whisk until the spices are evenly distributed.

5. **Simmer:**
    - Allow the hot chocolate to simmer for a few minutes, stirring occasionally. This helps the flavors meld together.

6. **Serve:**
    - Pour the spiced honey hot chocolate into mugs. If desired, top with whipped cream and a sprinkle of cinnamon.

7. **Enjoy:**
    - Sip and savor the comforting flavors of spiced honey hot chocolate!

Benefits of Spiced Honey Hot Chocolate:

1. **Antioxidant Properties:**
    - Cocoa powder is rich in antioxidants, which may help combat oxidative stress in the body.

2. **Immune Support (Honey):**
    - Honey has natural antibacterial and antioxidant properties that may contribute to overall immune support.

3. **Warmth and Comfort:**
    - The combination of spices, including cinnamon and nutmeg, adds warmth and comfort to the beverage, making it perfect for cold days or cozy evenings.

4. **Flavor Enhancement (Cayenne):**
   - A pinch of cayenne pepper can add a subtle kick to the hot chocolate, enhancing the overall flavor profile.

5. **Mood Booster:**
   - Enjoying a warm and indulgent beverage like spiced honey hot chocolate can contribute to a positive mood and a sense of well-being.

6. **Customizable:**
   - This recipe is highly customizable. You can adjust the sweetness, spice levels, or even experiment with different types of milk for a personalized experience.

7. **Hydration (Milk):**
   - Milk provides hydration and a source of essential nutrients like calcium and vitamin D.

8. **Optional Whipped Cream (Indulgence):**
   - Adding whipped cream is optional but adds a layer of indulgence to the drink.

Remember to tailor the recipe to your preferences and dietary needs. Whether you're looking for a sweet treat, a mood booster, or a comforting beverage, spiced honey hot chocolate is a versatile and delicious option.

Understanding honey bees.

Honey bees (Apis mellifera) are highly social insects known for their crucial role in pollination and honey production. Here are some key aspects to understand about honey bees:

Social Structure:

1. **Colony Organization:**
   - Honey bees live in colonies, which consist of three primary castes: the queen, worker bees, and drones.
2. **Queen Bee:**
   - There is only one queen in a hive. Her primary role is to lay eggs and maintain the colony. The queen is larger than other bees and can live for several years.
3. **Worker Bees:**
   - Worker bees are female and constitute the majority of the colony. They perform various tasks such as foraging, nursing, cleaning, and defending the hive. Worker bees live for a few weeks to a few months.
4. **Drones:**
   - Drones are male bees. Their primary role is to mate with a virgin queen during her nuptial flight. Drones do not have stingers and have a relatively short lifespan.

Life Cycle:

1. **Egg Stage:**
   - The queen lays eggs in individual cells of the comb. The eggs hatch into larvae.
2. **Larva Stage:**
   - Larvae are fed by worker bees and undergo several molting stages before pupation.
3. **Pupa Stage:**
   - The larvae spin a cocoon and transform into pupae, undergoing metamorphosis within the cell.
4. **Adult Stage:**
   - After completing development, an adult bee emerges from the cell.

Communication:

1. **Dances:**
   - Honey bees communicate with each other through intricate dances. The waggle dance indicates the direction and distance to a food source.
2. **Pheromones:**
   - Bees release pheromones to communicate various messages, such as marking the entrance of the hive or signaling danger.

Foraging and Pollination:

1. **Floral Preferences:**
   - Honey bees visit flowers to collect nectar, which they use to make honey. They also collect pollen for protein and other nutrients.
2. **Pollination:**
   - Honey bees are crucial pollinators for many flowering plants, including crops. They play a vital role in agriculture by facilitating the reproduction of plants.

Hive Products:

1. **Honey:**
   - Honey bees produce honey by collecting nectar from flowers, which they transform and store in the hive.
2. **Beeswax:**
   - Beeswax is secreted by worker bees and used to build comb for honey storage and as a platform for raising brood.
3. **Royal Jelly:**
   - Worker bees produce royal jelly to feed larvae. It is also used to feed the queen throughout her life.

Threats and Challenges:

1. **Pesticides:**

- Exposure to pesticides poses a significant threat to honey bee populations.

2. **Parasites and Diseases:**
   - Varroa mites and diseases like Nosema can weaken and decimate bee colonies.

3. **Loss of Habitat:**
   - Changes in land use and loss of natural habitats impact foraging opportunities for bees.

Conservation and Beekeeping:

1. **Beekeeping:**
   - Beekeepers manage hives to harvest honey, beeswax, and other hive products. Responsible beekeeping practices contribute to pollinator health.

2. **Conservation Efforts:**
   - Conservation initiatives focus on protecting and restoring habitats, reducing pesticide use, and raising awareness about the importance of bees.

Understanding honey bees is crucial for promoting their well-being and ensuring their vital role in ecosystems and agriculture. Bee conservation efforts are essential to address the challenges facing bee populations worldwide.

What herbs can I use as an antibiotic?

Several herbs are known for their potential antibiotic properties, offering natural alternatives to synthetic antibiotics. Keep in mind that while some herbs may possess antibacterial properties, they may not replace prescribed antibiotics in severe bacterial infections. Always consult with a healthcare professional before using herbs for medicinal purposes. Here are some herbs with antibiotic properties:

1. **Garlic (Allium sativum):**
   - Garlic contains allicin, a compound with antimicrobial properties. It has been used traditionally to fight infections and boost the immune system.
2. **Oregano (Origanum vulgare):**
   - Oregano oil has demonstrated antibacterial, antiviral, and antifungal properties. It contains compounds such as carvacrol and thymol.
3. **Turmeric (Curcuma longa):**
   - Curcumin, the active compound in turmeric, exhibits antibacterial and anti-inflammatory properties. It has been used in traditional medicine for various health benefits.
4. **Echinacea (Echinacea purpurea):**

- Echinacea is known for its immune-boosting properties. It may help the body fight off infections, and some studies suggest it has antimicrobial effects.

5. **Ginger (Zingiber officinale):**
    - Ginger has antimicrobial and anti-inflammatory properties. It has been used in traditional medicine to combat infections and soothe various ailments.

6. **Goldenseal (Hydrastis canadensis):**
    - Goldenseal contains berberine, a compound with antibacterial and anti-inflammatory properties. It has been used traditionally to treat infections.

7. **Thyme (Thymus vulgaris):**
    - Thyme contains thymol, a natural compound with antimicrobial properties. Thyme oil has been used for its antibacterial and antifungal effects.

8. **Manuka Honey:**
    - Manuka honey, produced in New Zealand, has potent antibacterial properties. It is used topically to promote wound healing and fight infections.

9. **Cinnamon (Cinnamomum verum):**
    - Cinnamon has antimicrobial properties, and its essential oil has been studied for its ability to inhibit the growth of bacteria.

10. **Neem (Azadirachta indica):**

- Neem has been used in traditional medicine for its antibacterial, antiviral, and antifungal properties. It is often used topically for skin conditions.

11. **Andrographis (Andrographis paniculata):**
    - Andrographis has been used in traditional medicine for its immune-boosting and antibacterial properties.

It's important to note that the efficacy of herbs can vary, and individual responses may differ. Additionally, if you are considering using herbs for medicinal purposes, especially as an alternative to antibiotics, it's crucial to consult with a healthcare professional. They can provide guidance based on your specific health condition, ensuring safe and effective use.

What are some health benefits of garlic? How do you use it?

Garlic (Allium sativum) is not only a flavorful culinary ingredient but also has a long history of being valued for its potential health benefits. Here are some health benefits of garlic and ways to incorporate it into your diet:

Health Benefits of Garlic:

1. **Antimicrobial Properties:**
   - Garlic possesses antimicrobial properties, including antibacterial, antiviral, and antifungal effects. It may help combat various infections.
2. **Heart Health:**
   - Garlic has been linked to cardiovascular benefits, including the potential to lower blood pressure and reduce cholesterol levels. It may also have anti-clotting effects.
3. **Anti-Inflammatory Effects:**
   - Compounds in garlic, such as allicin, have anti-inflammatory properties that may help reduce inflammation in the body.
4. **Immune System Support:**
   - Garlic is known for its immune-boosting properties. It may help enhance the immune system's ability to fight off infections and illnesses.
5. **Rich in Antioxidants:**
   - Garlic contains antioxidants that help protect cells from oxidative damage caused by free radicals. Antioxidants play a role in overall health and aging.
6. **Cancer Prevention:**
   - Some studies suggest that garlic may have cancer-fighting properties, particularly in relation to certain types of cancer, such as stomach and colorectal cancers.

7. **Improved Circulation:**
    - Garlic may help improve blood circulation, which can contribute to better overall vascular health.
8. **Detoxification:**
    - Garlic supports the body's natural detoxification processes and may help eliminate toxins.
9. **Anti-diabetic Effects:**
    - Garlic may have benefits for individuals with diabetes by helping regulate blood sugar levels.
10. **Respiratory Health:**
    - Garlic has been used traditionally to alleviate respiratory conditions. It may help in managing symptoms of common respiratory illnesses.

How to Use Garlic:

1. **Raw Garlic:**
    - Consuming raw garlic provides the maximum health benefits. You can add minced or crushed garlic to salads, dressings, or dips.
2. **Cooked Garlic:**
    - Incorporate garlic into cooked dishes like soups, stews, stir-fries, sauces, and roasted vegetables.

3. **Garlic Supplements:**
   - Garlic supplements, including garlic extract or garlic oil capsules, are available. However, it's important to consult with a healthcare professional before taking supplements.
4. **Garlic Tea:**
   - Make garlic tea by steeping crushed garlic in hot water. You can add honey and lemon for flavor.
5. **Fermented Garlic:**
   - Fermented garlic is a milder option. Fermentation may also enhance certain nutritional aspects.
6. **Garlic Oil:**
   - Use garlic-infused oil in cooking or as a drizzle for dishes like pasta, bread, or salads.
7. **Pickled Garlic:**
   - Pickled garlic provides a tangy flavor and can be enjoyed on its own or added to various dishes.
8. **Garlic-Rich Sauces:**
   - Create garlic-rich sauces, such as garlic butter, garlic aioli, or garlic-infused olive oil, to enhance the flavor of your meals.

Tips:

- **Let it Rest:**
  - After chopping or crushing garlic, let it sit for a few minutes before cooking to allow the formation of allicin, the beneficial compound responsible for many health benefits.
- **Moderation:**
  - While garlic is generally safe for most people, consuming excessive amounts may cause digestive discomfort for some individuals.
- **Consult a Professional:**
  - If you have specific health concerns or are taking medications, consult with a healthcare professional before incorporating large quantities of garlic into your diet or using garlic supplements.

Including garlic in your diet can be a flavorful and healthful addition, contributing to overall well-being.

What are the herbal remedies of turmeric? How do you use it?

Turmeric (Curcuma longa) is a popular spice that has been used for centuries in traditional medicine for its potential health benefits. The active compound in turmeric, curcumin, is known for its anti-inflammatory and antioxidant properties. Here are some herbal remedies and ways to use turmeric:

Herbal Remedies of Turmeric:

1. **Anti-Inflammatory Support:**
   - Turmeric is widely recognized for its anti-inflammatory effects. It may be beneficial in managing conditions associated with inflammation, such as arthritis. You can incorporate turmeric into your diet or consider turmeric supplements.
2. **Digestive Health:**
   - Turmeric may help support digestive health. It can be added to dishes or taken in supplement form. Some people use turmeric tea to ease digestive discomfort.
3. **Joint Pain Relief:**
   - Turmeric's anti-inflammatory properties may provide relief for joint pain. Turmeric supplements or incorporating turmeric into your diet may be helpful.
4. **Wound Healing:**
   - Turmeric has been traditionally used topically to aid in wound healing. A paste made from turmeric and water or turmeric-infused oil can be applied to minor cuts and wounds.
5. **Skin Conditions:**

- Turmeric may be beneficial for various skin conditions due to its anti-inflammatory and antioxidant properties. Turmeric paste or turmeric-infused oils can be applied to the skin.

6. **Immune System Support:**
   - Curcumin, the active compound in turmeric, has been studied for its potential immune-modulating effects. Including turmeric in your diet may contribute to overall immune system support.

7. **Antioxidant Boost:**
   - Turmeric is rich in antioxidants that help neutralize free radicals in the body. This may contribute to overall health and well-being.

How to Use Turmeric:

1. **Golden Milk (Turmeric Latte):**
   - Make a warm beverage known as golden milk by combining turmeric with milk (dairy or plant-based), a sweetener like honey, and optional spices such as ginger and cinnamon.

2. **Curries and Stews:**
   - Turmeric is a key ingredient in many curry dishes. Use it to flavor stews, soups, and other savory recipes.

3. **Turmeric Tea:**
   - Brew turmeric tea by steeping turmeric powder or fresh turmeric slices in hot water. Add lemon or honey for flavor.

4. **Smoothies:**
   - Add a pinch of turmeric powder or a small piece of fresh turmeric to your smoothies for an antioxidant boost.

5. **Turmeric Supplements:**
   - Turmeric supplements, often containing curcumin extract, are available in capsule or tablet form. Consult with a healthcare professional before taking supplements.

6. **Turmeric Paste:**
   - Make a turmeric paste by mixing turmeric powder with water. This paste can be applied topically to the skin or used in cooking.

7. **Turmeric Infused Oil:**
   - Create turmeric-infused oil by simmering turmeric in a carrier oil (such as coconut or olive oil). Use this oil topically or in cooking.

8. **Turmeric Face Mask:**
   - Mix turmeric with yogurt, honey, or aloe vera gel to create a face mask. Apply it to the face, leave it on for about 10-15 minutes, and then rinse off.

Tips:

- **Black Pepper Synergy:**
    - Consuming turmeric with black pepper enhances the absorption of curcumin, the active compound in turmeric. Piperine, a compound in black pepper, facilitates better absorption.
- **Stain Potential:**
    - Turmeric can stain surfaces and fabrics, so use caution when handling it.
- **Consult a Professional:**
    - If you are considering using turmeric for medicinal purposes or have existing health conditions, consult with a healthcare professional for personalized advice.

Turmeric is a versatile spice with a range of potential health benefits. Whether used in cooking, as a tea, or in topical applications, turmeric can be a valuable addition to a health-conscious lifestyle.

What are the health benefits of echinacea? How do you use it?

Echinacea, commonly known as purple coneflower, is a flowering plant native to North America. It has been used traditionally in Native American herbal medicine, and today, it is popularly used as a supplement for various health purposes. Here are some potential health benefits of echinacea and ways to use it:

Health Benefits of Echinacea:

1. **Immune System Support:**
   - Echinacea is often used to support the immune system. It may help stimulate the production of white blood cells and enhance the body's defense against infections.
2. **Cold and Flu Relief:**
   - Echinacea supplements or herbal teas are commonly used to alleviate symptoms of the common cold and flu. Some people take echinacea at the onset of symptoms for potential symptom reduction and faster recovery.
3. **Anti-Inflammatory Properties:**
   - Echinacea has anti-inflammatory properties, which may contribute to its immune-modulating effects. It could be beneficial for conditions involving inflammation.
4. **Wound Healing:**
   - Echinacea has been used topically to promote wound healing. Creams or ointments containing echinacea extracts

may be applied to minor cuts, burns, or skin irritations.

5. **Respiratory Health:**
   - Echinacea is sometimes used to support respiratory health, particularly in addressing conditions such as bronchitis or sinusitis.

6. **Antioxidant Activity:**
   - Echinacea contains compounds with antioxidant properties, helping neutralize free radicals in the body and potentially supporting overall health.

How to Use Echinacea:

1. **Echinacea Tea:**
   - Echinacea tea is a popular and easy way to consume echinacea. You can find echinacea tea bags or use dried echinacea roots or flowers to make your own tea. Steep in hot water for about 5-10 minutes before drinking.

2. **Echinacea Supplements:**
   - Echinacea is available in various supplement forms, including capsules, tablets, and tinctures. Follow the recommended dosage on the product label, and consult with a healthcare professional before using supplements.

3. **Echinacea Tinctures:**

- Echinacea tinctures are liquid extracts that can be taken sublingually (under the tongue) or added to water. Tinctures provide a concentrated form of echinacea.

4. **Echinacea Capsules or Tablets:**
   - Capsules or tablets containing echinacea extract are convenient for those who prefer a standardized dosage.

5. **Echinacea in Food:**
   - While echinacea is not commonly used in cooking, you may find some herbal recipes that include echinacea flowers or roots. Keep in mind that heating may reduce the potency of certain compounds.

6. **Topical Echinacea Preparations:**
   - Echinacea creams, ointments, or salves are available for topical application. These may be used on minor wounds, cuts, or skin irritations.

Tips:

- **Quality Matters:**
  - When choosing echinacea supplements, opt for reputable brands to ensure the product contains the stated amount of active compounds.
- **Consult a Healthcare Professional:**

- If you are pregnant, breastfeeding, have allergies, or are taking medications, consult with a healthcare professional before using echinacea supplements.
- **Short-Term Use:**
  - Echinacea is often recommended for short-term use, such as during the onset of cold symptoms. Prolonged use may diminish its effectiveness.
- **Individual Responses Vary:**
  - Echinacea's effectiveness can vary among individuals. Some people may experience benefits, while others may not respond as significantly.

It's important to note that while echinacea is generally considered safe for most people, individual responses can vary, and it may not be suitable for everyone. As with any herbal supplement, it's advisable to consult with a healthcare professional before incorporating echinacea into your routine, especially if you have underlying health conditions or are taking medications.

What is goldenseal? Does it come in a capsule? How do you use it and what are the herbal remedies for it?

Goldenseal (Hydrastis canadensis) is a perennial herb native to the eastern United States and Canada. It has a long history of use in traditional Native American medicine and later became a popular herb in Western herbalism. The root of the goldenseal plant is primarily used for its medicinal properties. Here's an overview of goldenseal, its forms, uses, and herbal remedies:

Goldenseal Overview:

1. **Active Compounds:**
   - Goldenseal contains various alkaloids, including berberine, hydrastine, and canadine. Berberine is a key compound associated with many of its health benefits.
2. **Traditional Uses:**
   - Goldenseal has been traditionally used for its potential antimicrobial, anti-inflammatory, and immune-enhancing properties.
3. **Forms:**
   - Goldenseal is available in different forms, including:
     - **Capsules or Tablets:** These are convenient for standardized dosages.
     - **Liquid Extracts or Tinctures:** These provide a concentrated liquid form.

- **Powders:** Ground goldenseal root is available as a powder for teas or other preparations.

Herbal Remedies and Uses:

1. **Immune Support:**
   - Goldenseal is believed to support the immune system. It has been historically used to address respiratory infections and seasonal illnesses.
2. **Antimicrobial Properties:**
   - Berberine, a key compound in goldenseal, has demonstrated antimicrobial effects. Goldenseal has been used to address various infections, including bacterial and fungal infections.
3. **Digestive Health:**
   - Goldenseal may support digestive health and has been used traditionally for conditions like diarrhea and indigestion.
4. **Topical Uses:**
   - External preparations with goldenseal, such as creams or ointments, have been used for skin conditions, wounds, and eye infections.
5. **Mucous Membrane Support:**
   - Goldenseal has astringent properties that may support mucous membrane health. It has been used for conditions affecting the

mucous membranes, such as sinus congestion.

How to Use Goldenseal:

1. **Capsules or Tablets:**
   - Goldenseal supplements in capsule or tablet form are a convenient way to take standardized doses. Follow the recommended dosage on the product label.
2. **Liquid Extracts or Tinctures:**
   - Liquid extracts provide a concentrated form of goldenseal. They can be taken directly or diluted in water or juice. Follow the recommended dosage.
3. **Tea:**
   - You can prepare goldenseal tea using the dried root powder. Steep the powder in hot water for about 10 minutes, strain, and drink. Note that the taste can be bitter.
4. **Topical Preparations:**
   - Creams, ointments, or salves containing goldenseal can be applied topically to the skin for wound healing or addressing skin conditions.

Tips:

- **Quality and Dosage:**
    - Choose reputable brands for goldenseal supplements to ensure quality. Follow recommended dosages and consult with a healthcare professional if unsure.
- **Consult a Professional:**
    - If you are pregnant, breastfeeding, or taking medications, consult with a healthcare professional before using goldenseal supplements.
- **Short-Term Use:**
    - Goldenseal is often recommended for short-term use due to concerns about overharvesting and potential side effects with prolonged use.
- **Combine with Echinacea:**
    - Goldenseal is sometimes combined with echinacea for immune support, creating herbal blends.

It's crucial to approach the use of goldenseal with caution, considering individual health conditions and potential interactions with medications. While it has a history of traditional use, scientific evidence supporting some of its uses is limited, and more research is needed to fully understand its effectiveness and safety. As with any herbal supplement, consulting with a healthcare professional is advisable before use.

What are the herbal remedies for thyme? How do you use it? Does it come in a capsule or is it better natural?

Thyme (Thymus vulgaris) is a fragrant herb that has been used for both culinary and medicinal purposes for centuries. It contains various compounds, including thymol, which contributes to its potential health benefits. Here are some herbal remedies for thyme and ways to use it:

Herbal Remedies for Thyme:

1. **Respiratory Health:**
   - Thyme has long been used to support respiratory health. It may help relieve symptoms of coughs, colds, and bronchitis. Thyme tea or steam inhalation with thyme essential oil can be beneficial.
2. **Antimicrobial Properties:**
   - Thyme exhibits antimicrobial properties, including antibacterial and antifungal effects. It may be used for throat infections, as a mouthwash, or for minor skin irritations.
3. **Digestive Aid:**
   - Thyme can be used to promote digestive health. It may help with indigestion, bloating, and gas. Thyme tea or adding

fresh thyme to meals are common methods.

4. **Anti-Inflammatory Effects:**
   - Thyme contains anti-inflammatory compounds that may be beneficial for conditions associated with inflammation. Thyme tea or incorporating thyme into dishes may contribute to overall health.

5. **Boosting Immunity:**
   - Thyme has immune-boosting properties due to its antioxidant content. Regular consumption, such as in thyme tea, may support the immune system.

How to Use Thyme:

1. **Thyme Tea:**
   - Prepare thyme tea by steeping fresh or dried thyme leaves in hot water for about 5-10 minutes. Strain and drink. Add honey or lemon for flavor if desired.

2. **Culinary Uses:**
   - Incorporate fresh or dried thyme into your cooking. It pairs well with a variety of dishes, including soups, stews, roasted vegetables, and meats.

3. **Thyme Infusions:**
   - Create thyme-infused oils or vinegars for culinary use. These infusions can be made

by steeping thyme in oil or vinegar over time.

4. **Thyme Essential Oil:**
   - Thyme essential oil is potent and should be used with caution. It can be diffused for aromatherapy or diluted and applied topically for various purposes. Consult with a qualified aromatherapist or healthcare professional for guidance.

Thyme Supplements:

While thyme supplements in the form of capsules or tablets are less common than culinary or tea use, they do exist. However, the benefits of thyme are often best obtained through natural forms, as the combination of various compounds in the whole herb may contribute to its effectiveness. If considering thyme supplements, choose reputable brands, and consult with a healthcare professional before use, especially if you have any existing health conditions or are taking medications.

Tips:

- **Fresh vs. Dried Thyme:**
  - Both fresh and dried thyme can be used, but their flavors may differ. Fresh thyme is often preferred in salads and garnishes, while dried thyme is convenient for cooking.

- **Consult a Professional:**
  - If you are pregnant, breastfeeding, or have health concerns, consult with a healthcare professional before using thyme in medicinal quantities.
- **Consider Culinary Uses:**
  - Incorporating thyme into your meals not only adds flavor but also provides potential health benefits.
- **Moderation:**
  - While thyme is generally safe when used in culinary amounts, using excessive amounts or concentrated forms like essential oil may have adverse effects. Use moderation and seek guidance if needed.

Thyme, in its various forms, can be a versatile and healthful addition to both your culinary repertoire and your herbal medicine cabinet. As with any herb or supplement, individual responses may vary, and it's advisable to seek guidance from a healthcare professional if you have specific health concerns or questions.

What are the natural remedies for cinnamon? How do you use it? Are there cinnamon capsules or do you use it naturally?

Cinnamon (Cinnamomum verum or Cinnamomum cassia) is a widely used spice known for its sweet and warm flavor. In addition to its culinary uses, cinnamon has been studied for its potential health benefits, and it has a history of use in traditional medicine. Here are some natural remedies for cinnamon and ways to use it:

Natural Remedies for Cinnamon:

1. **Blood Sugar Regulation:**
   - Cinnamon may help improve insulin sensitivity and contribute to better blood sugar control. Regular consumption, particularly of Ceylon cinnamon, has been studied for its potential benefits in individuals with diabetes or insulin resistance.
2. **Anti-Inflammatory Effects:**
   - Cinnamon contains compounds with anti-inflammatory properties. It may be used to alleviate inflammation associated with various conditions.
3. **Antioxidant Properties:**
   - Cinnamon is rich in antioxidants, which help neutralize free radicals in the body. Antioxidants play a role in overall health and may contribute to aging well.
4. **Heart Health:**

- Some studies suggest that cinnamon may have positive effects on heart health by helping to lower cholesterol levels and blood pressure.

5. **Digestive Health:**
   - Cinnamon has been used traditionally to aid digestion. It may help alleviate indigestion, bloating, and gas.

6. **Anti-Microbial Properties:**
   - Cinnamon exhibits antimicrobial properties, which may help combat bacteria and fungi. It can be used topically or as part of oral care routines.

How to Use Cinnamon:

1. **Culinary Uses:**
   - Incorporate cinnamon into your diet through various culinary applications. Add it to oatmeal, yogurt, smoothies, baked goods, and hot beverages like tea or coffee.

2. **Cinnamon Tea:**
   - Make cinnamon tea by steeping a cinnamon stick or ground cinnamon in hot water. You can add honey or lemon for flavor.

3. **Cinnamon Water Infusions:**

- Infuse water with cinnamon by adding cinnamon sticks to a pitcher of water. Refrigerate and enjoy cinnamon-infused water throughout the day.

4. **Topical Applications:**

    - Create a paste by mixing cinnamon with honey and use it topically for minor skin irritations or as a face mask.

Cinnamon Supplements:

Cinnamon supplements, including capsules or extracts, are available. However, the efficacy of supplements can vary, and it's essential to choose high-quality products. Before considering cinnamon supplements, especially in higher concentrations, consult with a healthcare professional, particularly if you have any existing health conditions or are taking medications.

Tips:

- **Type of Cinnamon:**
    - There are different types of cinnamon, with Ceylon and Cassia being the most common. Ceylon cinnamon is considered "true" or "sweet" cinnamon and is generally recommended for regular use due to lower coumarin levels, especially for those using cinnamon in larger quantities.
- **Moderation:**

- While cinnamon is generally safe when used in culinary amounts, excessive intake of cinnamon supplements may have adverse effects. Use moderation and follow recommended dosages.
- **Consult a Professional:**
  - If you have diabetes or any existing health conditions, consult with a healthcare professional before incorporating cinnamon supplements into your routine.

Cinnamon is a versatile spice that can be easily incorporated into your daily routine. Whether used in cooking or consumed as a tea, cinnamon can contribute not only to the flavor of your dishes but also to potential health benefits. Always approach the use of supplements with caution and seek guidance from a healthcare professional if needed.

What is neem? How do you use it as a natural remedy?

Neem (Azadirachta indica) is a tree native to the Indian subcontinent and is known for its various medicinal properties. All parts of the neem tree, including the leaves, bark, seeds, and oil, have been traditionally used in Ayurvedic medicine for their therapeutic benefits.

Here are some aspects of neem and how it is used as a natural remedy:

Neem Components:

1. **Neem Leaves:**
   - Neem leaves are rich in compounds like nimbin, nimbidin, and nimbidol. They are often used for their antibacterial, antiviral, and antifungal properties.
2. **Neem Bark:**
   - The bark of the neem tree contains compounds such as tannins and flavonoids, which contribute to its anti-inflammatory and antioxidant effects.
3. **Neem Seeds:**
   - Neem seeds are a source of neem oil, which is known for its pesticidal properties and is also used in skincare products.

Natural Remedies Using Neem:

1. **Skin Conditions:**
   - Neem has been traditionally used to address various skin issues. Neem oil or a paste made from neem leaves can be applied topically to soothe conditions like acne, eczema, psoriasis, and fungal infections.

2. **Oral Health:**
   - Neem has natural antibacterial properties that make it beneficial for oral health. Chewing neem twigs or using neem-based toothpaste may help reduce bacteria in the mouth, preventing issues like gum disease and cavities.
3. **Immune Support:**
   - Neem is believed to have immune-boosting properties. Consuming neem extracts or infusions may contribute to overall immune system support.
4. **Insect Repellent:**
   - Neem oil is known for its insect-repelling properties. It can be used as a natural alternative to chemical insecticides for controlling pests in gardens or on plants.
5. **Hair Care:**
   - Neem oil is used in hair care products for its potential to improve scalp health, reduce dandruff, and promote hair growth. It can be applied to the scalp or added to hair care formulations.
6. **Digestive Health:**
   - Neem extracts may have benefits for digestive health. Neem leaves or neem supplements may be consumed to support gastrointestinal well-being.

How to Use Neem:

1. **Neem Oil:**
   - Neem oil can be applied topically to the skin or added to shampoos and conditioners for hair care. It can also be diluted and used as a natural insect repellent.
2. **Neem Leaf Paste:**
   - Make a paste by grinding neem leaves and applying it to affected areas of the skin. This can be helpful for addressing skin conditions.
3. **Neem Tea:**
   - Infuse neem leaves in hot water to make neem tea. This tea can be consumed for potential immune support or digestive benefits.
4. **Neem Chewing Sticks:**
   - Neem twigs or chewing sticks are traditionally used for oral care. Chewing on these sticks is believed to promote oral hygiene.
5. **Neem Capsules or Supplements:**
   - Neem is available in supplement form, such as capsules or tablets. Consult with a healthcare professional before using neem supplements, especially in higher concentrations.

Tips:

- **Consult a Professional:**
    - If you are pregnant, breastfeeding, or have health concerns, consult with a healthcare professional before using neem as a remedy.
- **Patch Test:**
    - Before applying neem oil or paste to a larger area of the skin, conduct a patch test to ensure you do not have an allergic reaction.
- **Use Caution with Neem Oil:**
    - Neem oil is potent, and using excessive amounts may cause skin irritation. Always follow recommended dilution guidelines.

Neem offers a range of potential health benefits, and its versatility makes it suitable for various applications. While neem is generally safe for external use and traditional consumption in culinary amounts, it's important to approach its use with caution, especially in concentrated forms. If you have specific health concerns or questions, consulting with a healthcare professional is advisable.

What are the benefits of honey for women?

Honey offers a variety of potential health benefits for women, ranging from general well-being to specific aspects of women's health. Here are some potential benefits of honey for women:

General Health:

1. **Energy Boost:**
   - The natural sugars in honey, primarily fructose and glucose, provide a quick energy boost. This can be beneficial for women with busy schedules or those engaging in physical activities.
2. **Antioxidant Properties:**
   - Honey contains antioxidants that help neutralize free radicals in the body. Antioxidants contribute to overall health and may have anti-aging effects.
3. **Immune Support:**
   - Honey's antibacterial and antimicrobial properties may support the immune system, helping women ward off common illnesses.
4. **Digestive Health:**
   - Honey is believed to have digestive benefits. Consuming honey, particularly raw honey, may help soothe the digestive tract and alleviate symptoms like indigestion.

Women's Health:

5. **Soothing Menstrual Symptoms:**
   - Some women find relief from menstrual symptoms by incorporating honey into their diet. Warm honey mixed with herbal teas or warm water may provide soothing effects.
6. **Skin Care:**
   - Honey's natural antibacterial properties can be beneficial for skin health. Women may use honey in homemade face masks or skin care routines to promote a healthy complexion.
7. **Cough and Sore Throat Relief:**
   - Honey is known for its soothing effects on the throat. Women experiencing coughs or sore throats may find relief by consuming honey or adding it to warm beverages.
8. **Wound Healing:**
   - Honey has been used for wound healing and may be applied topically to minor cuts or abrasions. Its antimicrobial properties may help prevent infection.
9. **Preventing Urinary Tract Infections (UTIs):**
   - Some studies suggest that honey may have antibacterial effects that could be helpful in preventing urinary tract infections.

However, more research is needed in this area.

Culinary Uses:

10. **Natural Sweetener:**
    - Honey can be used as a natural sweetener in a variety of dishes, offering a healthier alternative to refined sugars.
11. **Flavor Enhancer:**
    - Incorporating honey into recipes can enhance flavors, making it a versatile ingredient in both sweet and savory dishes.

Tips:

- **Choose Raw Honey:**
    - Raw honey retains more of its natural nutrients and antioxidants compared to processed honey. When possible, choose raw, unfiltered honey for maximum benefits.
- **Moderation is Key:**
    - While honey offers health benefits, it's important to consume it in moderation due to its high sugar content. Excessive sugar intake may have negative effects on health.
- **Consult a Professional:**

- If you have specific health concerns or conditions, consult with a healthcare professional for personalized advice on incorporating honey into your diet.

It's important to note that individual responses to honey can vary, and some benefits may be anecdotal. As with any dietary changes or additions, it's advisable for women to consult with a healthcare professional, especially if they have existing health conditions or concerns.

What are the benefits of honey to men?

Honey offers several potential health benefits for men, contributing to overall well-being and addressing specific health concerns. Here are some benefits of honey for men:

General Health:

1. **Energy Boost:**
   - The natural sugars in honey, such as fructose and glucose, provide a quick energy boost. This can be particularly beneficial for men with active lifestyles or those engaging in physical activities.
2. **Antioxidant Properties:**

- Honey contains antioxidants that help neutralize free radicals in the body. Antioxidants contribute to overall health, supporting the body's defense against oxidative stress.

3. **Immune Support:**
   - The antibacterial and antimicrobial properties of honey may help support the immune system, assisting in preventing common illnesses.

4. **Digestive Health:**
   - Honey is believed to have digestive benefits. Consuming honey, especially raw honey, may help soothe the digestive tract and alleviate symptoms like indigestion.

Men's Health:

5. **Prostate Health:**
   - Some studies suggest that honey may have potential benefits for prostate health. Research in this area is ongoing, and more evidence is needed to establish a clear connection.

6. **Reproductive Health:**
   - Honey's antioxidant properties may contribute to reproductive health. Antioxidants help protect sperm from

oxidative stress, potentially benefiting male fertility.

7. **Soothing Cough and Sore Throat:**
   - Honey is known for its soothing effects on the throat. Men experiencing coughs or sore throats may find relief by consuming honey or adding it to warm beverages.

8. **Wound Healing:**
   - Honey has been used traditionally for wound healing. Its antimicrobial properties may help prevent infection, making it useful for treating minor cuts or abrasions.

Culinary Uses:

9. **Natural Sweetener:**
   - Honey can serve as a healthier alternative to refined sugars, acting as a natural sweetener in various dishes.

10. **Flavor Enhancer:**
   - Incorporating honey into recipes can enhance flavors, making it a versatile ingredient in both sweet and savory dishes.

Tips:

- **Choose Raw Honey:**

- Opt for raw, unfiltered honey when possible to maximize its natural nutrients and health benefits.
- **Moderation is Key:**
  - While honey is beneficial, it's important to consume it in moderation due to its high sugar content.
- **Consult a Professional:**
  - If there are specific health concerns or conditions, men should consult with a healthcare professional for personalized advice on incorporating honey into their diet.

Individual responses to honey can vary, and it's important to consider personal health conditions and dietary preferences. As with any dietary changes or additions, men should seek guidance from healthcare professionals, especially if they have existing health concerns.

What are 50 benefits of honey?

Honey is a versatile natural ingredient that offers numerous potential health benefits. While it's important to note that individual responses can vary, here are 50 potential benefits of honey:

General Health:

1. **Energy Boost:** Honey's natural sugars provide a quick energy boost.
2. **Antioxidant Support:** Rich in antioxidants, honey helps combat oxidative stress.
3. **Immune System Support:** Antibacterial properties may support the immune system.
4. **Cough Relief:** Soothes sore throats and provides cough relief.
5. **Digestive Aid:** May help soothe the digestive tract and alleviate indigestion.
6. **Wound Healing:** Antimicrobial properties make honey useful for wound healing.
7. **Improved Sleep:** A small amount of honey before bedtime may improve sleep quality.

Skin Health:

8. **Acne Treatment:** Honey's antibacterial properties can help with acne.
9. **Moisturizing Face Mask:** Used in face masks, honey moisturizes and nourishes the skin.
10. **Scar Reduction:** Applied topically, honey may reduce the appearance of scars.
11. **Anti-Aging Properties:** Antioxidants in honey contribute to anti-aging effects.
12. **Sunburn Relief:** Soothes sunburn and promotes healing.

Respiratory Health:

13. **Asthma Relief:** Honey may help soothe asthma symptoms.
14. **Sinus Infection Relief:** Combats bacteria and soothes sinus infections.
15. **Throat Infections:** Helps alleviate symptoms of throat infections.
16. **Seasonal Allergies:** Local honey may help with seasonal allergy symptoms.

Oral Health:

17. **Cavity Prevention:** Natural antibacterial properties may help prevent cavities.
18. **Gum Health:** Chewing on honeycomb or using honey-based products may support gum health.
19. **Bad Breath:** Natural sweeteners in honey may help combat bad breath.

Cardiovascular Health:

20. **Cholesterol Reduction:** Regular consumption may help lower cholesterol levels.
21. **Blood Pressure Regulation:** Some studies suggest honey may help regulate blood pressure.
22. **Heart Health:** Antioxidants in honey contribute to overall heart health.

Gastrointestinal Health:

23. **Ulcer Treatment:** Honey's antimicrobial properties may aid in treating ulcers.
24. **Constipation Relief:** Honey in warm water may help relieve constipation.
25. **Gastric Issues:** May help soothe and alleviate gastric issues.

Reproductive Health:

26. **Male Fertility:** Antioxidants in honey may contribute to male reproductive health.
27. **Female Fertility:** Some studies suggest honey may support female fertility.

Athletic Performance:

28. **Pre-Workout Energy:** Honey provides a natural energy boost for workouts.
29. **Post-Workout Recovery:** Natural sugars aid in post-exercise recovery.

Weight Management:

30. **Weight Loss Support:** Used as a natural sweetener, honey can be part of a balanced diet.

Diabetes Management:

31. **Moderate Glycemic Index:** Honey may have a lower impact on blood sugar levels than refined sugars.
32. **Insulin Sensitivity:** Some studies suggest honey may improve insulin sensitivity.

Psychological Well-Being:

33. **Stress Reduction:** Honey's natural sugars may help reduce stress.
34. **Improved Mood:** Natural sweeteners may contribute to improved mood.

Anti-Inflammatory Effects:

35. **Arthritis Relief:** Some people find honey helpful for reducing arthritis symptoms.
36. **Muscle Inflammation:** Honey may help reduce inflammation in muscles.

Hair Care:

37. **Scalp Health:** Honey in hair masks may improve scalp health.
38. **Dandruff Treatment:** Honey's antibacterial properties can help with dandruff.

Eye Health:

39. **Conjunctivitis Treatment:** Honey may be used in the treatment of conjunctivitis.

Respiratory Health:

40. **COPD Symptom Relief:** Some individuals report relief from COPD symptoms with honey.

Joint Health:

41. **Gout Management:** Honey may help manage symptoms of gout.

Pet Health:

42. **Wound Healing for Pets:** Honey may be used topically for pet wound healing.

Other Benefits:

43. **Natural Sweetener:** A healthier alternative to refined sugars.
44. **Hangover Relief:** Honey may help alleviate hangover symptoms.
45. **Eczema Relief:** Honey's antimicrobial properties may soothe eczema.
46. **Improved Cognitive Function:** Antioxidants in honey may support brain health.
47. **Improved Insulin Sensitivity:** Some studies suggest honey may improve insulin sensitivity.

48. **Alleviation of Allergic Reactions:** Local honey may help alleviate allergy symptoms.
49. **Liver Health:** Antioxidants in honey contribute to overall liver health.
50. **Anti-Cancer Properties:** Some studies suggest potential anti-cancer properties of honey, though more research is needed.

Tips:

- **Choose Raw Honey:** Opt for raw, unfiltered honey to retain maximum nutrients.
- **Moderation is Key:** Consume honey in moderation due to its high sugar content.
- **Consult a Professional:** Seek advice from healthcare professionals for specific health concerns or conditions.

While honey is generally considered safe for most people, it's important to consult with healthcare professionals, especially if you have specific health concerns or conditions. The benefits mentioned are based on anecdotal evidence and some scientific studies, and individual responses may vary.

In conclusion, this book has covered various aspects of honey, including its benefits for skin, hair, and health, as well as its use in recipes and beekeeping practices. We explored the diverse roles of honey, from its potential as a natural remedy to its significance in promoting overall well-being.

Key takeaways from this chat include:

1. **Health Benefits:** Honey offers a range of health benefits, serving as an antioxidant, antimicrobial agent, and potential contributor to heart health.
2. **Skin and Hair Care:** Honey can be beneficial for the skin, providing moisture and promoting wound healing. It may also be used in hair care routines.
3. **Nutritional Value:** While honey is a natural sweetener, it's important to use it in moderation due to its high sugar content. Raw and unprocessed honey retains more of its nutritional value.
4. **Beekeeping:** Building and maintaining beehives involve careful consideration of hive components, bee-friendly plants, and environmental factors to attract and support honeybee colonies.
5. **Recipes:** Honey is a versatile ingredient in various recipes, from beverages like honey lemonade to dishes like honey sesame roasted vegetables and honey walnut banana bread.

6. **Culinary Uses:** Honey serves as a natural sweetener and flavor enhancer in both sweet and savory dishes, contributing to a healthier alternative to refined sugars.

7. **Natural Remedies:** Honey has been used traditionally for its potential antibacterial and anti-inflammatory properties, making it a popular ingredient in home remedies.

Throughout this book, an emphasis was placed on the importance of sustainable and ethical beekeeping practices, as well as seeking advice from local experts for region-specific considerations.